nical Scenarios
Anaesthesia

For Churchill Livingstone

Commissioning Editor: Geoff Nuttall
Copy Editor: Susan Shatto
Project Controller: Elspett Masson
Design Direction: Sarah Cape

Clinical Scenarios in Anaesthesia

W. Alastair Chambers
Rona E. Patey

CHURCHILL LIVINGSTONE
EDINBURGH HONG KONG LONDON MADRID MELBOURNE
NEW YORK TOKYO 1995

CHURCHILL LIVINGSTONE
Medical Division of Pearson Professional Limited

Distributed in the United States of America by Churchill Livingstone Inc., 650 Avenue of the Americas, New York, N.Y. 1011, and by associated companies, branches and representatives throughout the world.

First published 1995

ISBN 0443 050708

British Library Cataloguing in Publication Data
A catalogue record for this book is available from the British Library.

Library of Congress Cataloging in Publication Data
A catalog record for this book is available from the Library of Congress.

The
publisher's
policy is to use
**paper manufactured
from sustainable forests**

Produced by Longman Singapore Publishers (Pte) Ltd.
Printed in Singapore

Contents

Preface

For the trainee in anaesthesia, much of the theoretical learning must of necessity be carried out in a structured manner and details of various techniques sought from some of the many excellent texts which are available. In the practical situation, cases do not arise in a neatly ordered fashion and many patients present with conditions which provide conflicting priorities.

Simulated clinical cases were introduced into the Part One examination to allow an assessment of the candidate's depth of knowledge in a more structured fashion than is possible in a clinical examination where 'live' patients are involved. The forthcoming changes in the examination structure have included changing the simulated clinical to the new final part of the fellowship examination. Clearly the scenarios which will be used will cover a much wider range of anaesthetic practice and the depth of knowledge expected will be much greater but the basic principles remain. The details of the case presented to the candidate will be fairly brief and the candidate will have a short time to consider the material and formulate a plan of action. The aims are to test the candidate's ability to develop and sustain a logical argument, to solve problems and apply factual knowledge to clinical situations and deal with complications which may be posed by the examiner. It is important to remember that there is seldom only one correct way to manage a given situation and it is vital to base answers on factual knowledge, to be able to defend a plan in the face of critical argument and to be aware of the merits and deficiencies of alternative actions.

This text aims to provide trainees in anaesthesia with a variety of problem cases and sets out to ask more questions than it answers. A wide variety of surgical specialties are represented but we have not attempted to include everything. The details given on nearly all cases is far in excess of that which would be presented in the examination as we felt that giving a fuller account of each case would give the reader more possibilities to consider. The conduct of the cases is not always the only or necessarily the best technique and the reader is invited to consider whether he or she would have acted differently. The important skill for the trainee to acquire is the ability to comment critically on a given case and to be prepared to defend their opinion. The scope of the text is deliberately short and no attempt has been made to fully consider every option. Recommendations for further reading are made for each case. The scenarios described are based on actual case histories although in many cases details have been amended in order to provide additional illustrative learning material.

Acknowledgements

We record our thanks to the following members of the Department of Anaesthetics at the Aberdeen Royal Hospitals NHS Trust who have contributed cases to this text: Fiona Bryden, Alison Campbell, Rob Casson, Michael Crawford, Graham Johnstone, Fiona Knox, Harry McFarlane, Paul Martin, John Read, Andrew Ronald, Donnie Ross and Michael Steyn.

We also wish to thank Prof Jamie Weir for assistance with the radiological illustrations.

W.A.C.
R.P.

1 Haematemesis

A 79-year-old woman presented to the on-call medical ward with a history of haematemesis that day and dark bowel motions for 3 days. The only finding of note in her past medical history was osteoarthritis, for which she took nonsteroidal anti-inflammatory drugs. She lived in sheltered housing, had a home help, but was otherwise self-caring.

On initial examination she was pale and sweaty, with a blood pressure of 100/50 mmHg and pulse rate of 129/min. Intravenous access was established and transfusion of crystalloid commenced after obtaining blood for full blood count, urea and electrolytes and the emergency cross-match of 4 units of packed red cells. This sample revealed the haemoglobin was 8 g/dl and urea was 14.5 mmol/l with other blood indices within normal limits. Chest X-ray showed a mild degree of cardiomegaly and ECG displayed sinus tachycardia with evidence of left ventricular hypertrophy.

Following infusion of one litre of crystalloid, the transfusion of blood commenced and she was taken for upper GI endoscopy. This was facilitated by the administration of midazolam intravenously. A gastric ulcer, with clot formation on the lesser curvature was seen, not actively bleeding. Conservative management was planned in view of her age and these findings. The blood transfusion continued, a urinary catheter was passed and intravenous ranitidine commenced. With this management her condition steadily improved, with heart rate and blood pressure returning to normal levels and urine output stabilising at 25 ml/h.

Six hours later she complained again of feeling unwell. Her pulse rate increased and blood pressure fell, and shortly after she passed a large maelena stool followed by further fresh haematemesis. A surgical opinion was sought. This was felt to be evidence of a second significant bleed, and it was decided she should undergo emergency laparotomy. A further 6 units of packed cells were cross-matched.

In the anaesthetic room basic monitoring was established revealing a heart rate of 128/min, blood pressure 90/59 mmHg and S_pO_2 94%. During 5 minutes of pre-oxygenation, 500 ml of crystalloid solution was infused through a 14 G cannula in one antecubital fossa and 400 ml of PPS through a 16 G cannula in the opposite forearm. The heart rate decreased to 115/min and blood pressure increased to 110/60 mmHg. Anaesthesia was induced with a rapid sequence intravenous technique using etomidate and suxamethonium. Anaesthesia was maintained with isoflurane and 50% nitrous oxide in oxygen. Morphine was given for analgesia and atracurium provided further muscle relaxation. A central line was inserted to the right internal jugular vein and a large-bore naso-gastric tube passed from which 300 ml of fresh blood were aspirated. Transfusion of warmed fluids continued, and an infusion of low-dose dopamine was commenced through the central line.

Surgery proceeded uneventfully. The gastric ulcer seen at endoscopy was confirmed and biopsied, then underrun and a vagotomy performed. By the end of the 90 minute procedure a further 4 units of packed red cells, 500 ml of crystalloid solution and 400 ml of PPS had been transfused at a rate sufficient to maintain a central venous pressure between 4 and 7 cmH$_2$O. Cardiovascular parameters were stable and 100 ml of urine was collected intra-operatively. Following reversal of neuromuscular blockade with neostigmine and glycopyrrolate and return of spontaneous ventilation, she was transferred on to her side into a warmed bed. When she opened her eyes to speech she was extubated and thereafter oxygen was administered via a Hudson mask. A patient controlled analgesia pump was connected in the recovery room, where she remained for 2 hours. On leaving the recovery room blood pressure was 145/85 mmHg, pulse rate 90/min, urine output greater than 15 ml each 30 min and the CVP was + 4 cm H$_2$O. A chest X-ray confirmed correct position of the central line. Her core temperature was 36.7°C. Intravenous infusion continued at 100 ml/h in the surgical high dependency unit overnight, with hourly urine volume and central venous pressure measurements.

DISCUSSION POINTS

This 79-year-old woman was independent and in good health before this admission. However, in the elderly there are changes in both body structure and function when compared to a young person, and a number of disease processes are increasingly common with increase in age.

● *Question 1: Outline the changes in the cardiovascular system expected with age, i.e. the disease processes commonly encountered, and discuss how these alter the ability to respond to fluid loss and fluid administration.*

- **Question 2:** *How might this influence the anaesthetic management of this type of case?*

Mortality following haematemesis remains significant.

- **Question 3:** *What guidelines exist for the management of this condition?*

- **Question 4:** *What factors would make you wish to consider surgical management?*

Renal function is altered significantly in the elderly, mainly due to changes in the renal vasculature. Up to 20% of the peri-operative mortality in elderly surgical patients has been reported as due to acute renal failure. This patient had evidence suggestive of renal dysfunction on admission (elevated urea), and her hypovolaemia constituted a significant renal insult. Low-dose dopamine is commonly used in patients thought to be at risk of renal dysfunction. However, there is little good clinical evidence available to suggest that dopamine has specific renal protective effects.

- **Question 5:** *Discuss the actions of dopamine on the renal system which have led to this widespread and continued use in the UK.*

- **Question 6:** *How would you optimize the condition of a patient presenting for major surgery with pre-operative renal dysfunction, and minimize the possibility of further renal insult?*

- **Question 7:** *Outline the factors in a patient's history, examination and pre-operative investigation which are associated with post-operative acute renal failure.*

This woman underwent upper gastro-intestinal endoscopy with the aid of intravenous midazolam.

- **Question 8:** *Comment on the use of sedative agents for this type of procedure, with particular reference to the problems which may occur and the type of monitoring which is suitable.*

This patient was nursed in the surgical high dependency unit postoperatively.

- **Question 9:** *Briefly consider if old age in itself is a contra-indication to ventilation and further resuscitation and monitoring in ITU.*

FURTHER READING

Muravchick S. Anaesthesia for the ageing patient. Can J Anaes 1993; 40: R63–68

Jones R M. Anaesthesia in old age. Anaesthesia 1989; 44: 337–8

Duke G J, Bersten A D. Dopamine and renal salvage in the critically ill patient. Anaesth Intensive Care 1992; 20: 277–302

Novis B K, Roizen M F, Aronston S, Thisted R A. Association of pre-operative risk factors with post-operative acute renal failure. Anes Analg 1994; 78: 143–149

Murray A W, Morran C G, Kenny G N C, MacFarlane P, Anderson J R. Examination of cardiorespiratory changes during upper gastrointestinal endoscopy. Anaesthesia 1991; 46: 181–4

O'Keefe S T, N. Chonchubhair A. Post-operative delirium in the elderly. Br J Anaes 1994; 673–687

2 Awareness

A 21-year-old 50 kg woman presented for an emergency appendicectomy. This was her first hospital admission and she was very anxious and in considerable discomfort. She had no past medical history of note. The anaesthetic SHO on call saw the woman on the ward and explained the proposed anaesthetic management to her. She thanked him and said she was reassured but still appeared anxious.

No premedication was given and on arrival in the anaesthetic room basic monitoring was established. Following pre-oxygenation, anaesthesia was induced using a rapid-sequence intravenous technique, with fentanyl, a sleep dose of thiopentone and suxamethonium. Cricoid pressure was applied and the trachea intubated with a cuffed orotracheal tube. The correct position of the tube was confirmed, cricoid pressure removed and maintenance of anaesthesia proceeded with enflurane 1.5% with 60% nitrous oxide in oxygen. The patient was then transferred to theatre. About 5 minutes after induction the patient was noted to cough and there was some movement of her limbs. Vecuronium was given. At surgery an inflamed appendix was found and removed. The procedure was straightforward and was completed 45 minutes after induction, whereupon anaesthesia was terminated and the neuromuscular blockade reversed with glycopyrrolate and neostigmine. Following establishment of spontaneous respiration and eye opening to speech she was extubated and taken to recovery, on her side, with oxygen 6L/min administered through a Hudson mask. Soon after her arrival there she received morphine 10 mg intramuscularly from the recovery room staff. The anaesthetist saw the patient in the recovery room 50 minutes later, when she was awake and comfortable.

The following day the anaesthetist was surprised to overhear nurses from the surgical ward discussing the patient and the fact that she claimed to have been aware of the incision and first few minutes of the operation. When he visited her in the ward, he found that this did indeed appear to be the case. She was tearful and demanded an explanation.

DISCUSSION POINTS

This instance of awareness was associated with pain, but other types of awareness have been described – for example: auditory with no pain; and amnesic awareness.

- *Question 1:* *Do all of these imply inadequate levels of anaesthesia? Do you know how commonly any of these occur?*

This patient had a rapid-sequence intravenous anaesthetic induction. This may be a time of particular risk of awareness.

- *Question 2:* *Why might this be, and what precautions could an anaesthetist take to reduce the risk safely?*

Anaesthesia requires an effective tension of the anaesthetic agent in the cerebral arterial blood.

- *Question 3:* *Which factors influence this? If you could monitor that tension, what would it guarantee about the level of consciousness in an individual?*

Classically, anaesthetists look for certain clinical signs that the patient is 'light'.

- *Question 4:* *Which signs are these? Are they a reliable guide to the depth of anaesthesia?*

The SHO in this instance went quickly to see the patient.

● *Question 5:* *Do you think he should have discussed this with his defence union before he did this? Is it likely his attitude to the patient might influence subsequent developments e.g., whether she proceeds to litigation?*

She may develop emotional or psychological problems as a result of this episode.

● *Question 6:* *What should the course of action be in this event?*

FURTHER READING

Depth of anaesthesia. Balliere's clinical anaesthesiology. vol 3, no 3. London: Balliere, 1989
Hargrove R L. Awareness under anaesthesia. Medical Defence Union 1987; 3: 9–11
Tunstall M E. The reduction of amnesic wakefulness during caesarean section. Anaesthesia 1979; 34: 316–9
McCrinick A, Evans G H, Thomas T A. Overpressure isoflurane at caesarean section: a study of arterial isoflurane concentrations. Br J Anaes 1994; 72: 122–4
Newton D E F. Awareness in anaesthesia. In: Atkinson R S, Adams A P, eds. Recent advances in anaesthesia and analgesia. 18th edn. Edinburgh: Churchill Livingstone, 1994
Cobcroft M D, Farsdick C. Awareness under anaesthesia: the patients' point of view. Anaesth and Intensive Care 1993; 21: 837–843

Ruptured aortic aneurysm

A 75-year-old man collapsed at home after developing severe back pain. His wife called the emergency service who brought him immediately to the Accident and Emergency Department. The paramedics reported that he was hypotensive (70/50 mmHg) with shallow respiration when they arrived at his home. Oxygen was commenced and an intravenous infusion established through which he received 500 ml normal saline during the 15 minute journey to hospital. On arrival, examination revealed a shocked patient with a pulsatile abdominal mass. A presumptive diagnosis of a leaking abdominal aortic aneurysm was made and the on-call vascular surgeon and anaesthetic team were informed.

Further intravenous access was established, blood was taken for urea and electrolyte measurement, full blood count and preparation of 10 units of type-specific blood. The patient was conscious, pale, sweaty and continued to complain of backache. His blood pressure was 100/60 mmHg and heart rate 110/min. One litre of gelatin solution was transfused. Past medical history obtained from his wife consisted of previous myocardial infarction, angina on climbing more than one flight of stairs and high blood pressure. Medications consisted of nifedipine, atenolol and GTN spray as required. He smoked 10 cigarettes per day. Twelve lead ECG showed evidence of a previous anterior myocardial infarction with lateral ischaemic changes. Chest X-ray was unremarkable. Results from the emergency blood samples were: haemoglobin, 12 g/dl; white cell count, $20 \times 10^{-9}/l$ and platelets 275; Na 140 mmol/l; K 3.9 mmol/l; urea 9.2 mmol/l; and creatinine 170 mmol/l. When the surgeon and anaesthetist arrived an abdominal ultrasound was performed. This confirmed the presence of aortic aneurysm, and in light of his shocked condition, immediate transfer to the emergency theatre was arranged.

On arrival in theatre blood pressure had fallen to 70/50 mmHg. Transfusion of two units of group O Rh negative blood was commenced. While the surgical staff scrubbed, arterial pressure monitoring via the right radial artery was established and a further large-bore intravenous cannula inserted. A urinary catheter was inserted as the patient was pre-oxygenated. There was no urine in the bladder. The patient was prepped and draped, then anaesthesia was induced with small increments of fentanyl and etomidate, followed by suxamethonium. The blood pressure was seen to fall from 100 mmHg to 60 mmHg. The trachea was intubated without difficulty and the patient ventilated with oxygen as the laparotomy commenced. Isoflurane was given at 0.2–0.6%, with atracurium to maintain neuromuscular blockade. Despite rapid infusion of fluid the systolic blood pressure remained 60 mmHg and the patient developed a supraventricular tachycardia of 180/min. The surgeons cross-clamped the aorta with difficulty. Despite this control of the bleeding and continued fluid administration, the tachycardia and hypotension persisted. Verapamil was given by slow intravenous injection. This reduced the heart rate to 120/min and the blood pressure rose to 90 mmHg systolic. Intravenous fluid administration continued peripherally as a 8.5FG sheath introducer was inserted into the right internal jugular vein. The CVP was measured as 25 mmHg. In light of this reading and the continued hypotension, dopamine was commenced.

After the patient was noted to have developed ischaemic ST segment changes on the ECG, a GTN infusion was commenced. A thermo-dilution pulmonary artery catheter was inserted. The capillary wedge pressure was measured as 20 mmHg and cardiac index calculated as 1.5 l/min/m^2. Blood pressure remained at 80–90 mmHg and the PCWP and CVP elevated despite the dopamine infusion. An adrenaline infusion was commenced, and the dopamine was decreased. The ECG continued to demonstrate an ischaemic pattern, and there was no urine output.

A straight vascular graft was inserted. Once this was complete (80 minutes after the start of the procedure with adrenaline, dopamine and GTN infusions continuing), the patient's heart rate was 125/min, blood pressure was 100/70 mmHg, CVP 20 mmHg, PCWP 18 mmHg and cardiac index 2.5 L/min/m^2. He had received 10 units of blood, 4 units of fresh frozen plasma, 1500 ml of other colloid and 1000 ml of crystalloid since his collapse. Measured blood loss was 4000 ml. Blood was sent for a clotting screen. When the cross-clamp was removed the blood pressure fell to 80 mmHg systolic. Blood gas measurement after cross-clamp release revealed a metabolic acidosis. Following administration of sodium bicarbonate and more fluid, the blood pressure rose to 110/80 mmHg. No urine had been passed since catheter insertion, so mannitol was given. He received 6 units of platelets once the results of the clotting screen were available.

After abdominal closure the patient was transferred to the intensive care unit for continued resuscitation, monitoring and ventilation. A 12-lead ECG suggested he had suffered an acute inferolateral myocardial infarction. He continued to be anuric despite high-dose diuretic administration and to require increasing inotropic support of his circulation.

DISCUSSION POINTS

Ruptured aortic aneurysm accounts for 0.5% of deaths in the general population. Whereas mortality from elective abdominal aneurysm repair is about 3%, mortality following emergency repair remains around 40%. Poor prognostic features include pre-operative hypotension, massive blood transfusion, myocardial impairment or cardiac arrest, poor urine output, and delays in diagnosis or prolonged surgery. Pre-operative factors such as increasing age, renal failure, ischaemic heart disease, hypertension and chronic obstructive airways disease are also associated with increased mortality.

There are two ways in which fluid resuscitation is managed pre-operatively in these patients. Classically, it has been said that intravenous fluid should be given to maintain an adequate blood pressure as systolic blood pressure is an indicator of survival. Alternatively, a lower blood pressure (systolic 50–70 mmHg) may be tolerated until the aorta is cross-clamped. Thereafter, fluid administration becomes maximal, to restore blood volume.

● *Question 1:* *Discuss the advantages and disadvantages of these two techniques.*

At least two anaesthetists are required to adequately manage this type of case. One to carry out continued resuscitation, the other to monitor the patient and administer anaesthesia. In this instance anaesthesia was induced once the surgeons were scrubbed and the field prepped and draped.

● *Question 2:* *Why was this? Outline a suitable anaesthetic technique for this procedure.*

ATLS training teaches peripheral venous cutdown in preference to central venous cannulation for initial administration of intravenous fluid in hypovolaemic traumatised patients. Some studies have shown subclavian vein cannulation to be quicker than basilic vein cut-down in experienced hands, with a similar complication rate.

● **Question 3:** *Discuss the factors determining fluid infusion rates, and the advantages and disadvantages of central and peripheral sites of cannulation.*

This case was associated with the transfusion of large amounts of fluid, much of it blood products. These fluids are inevitably cold. In addition, there are significant sources of heat loss in such a procedure.

● **Question 4:** *What are these sources and what measures might one take to counteract hypothermia?*

The patient suffered a myocardial infarction during surgery and required inotropic support.

● **Question 5:** *Describe other inotropes which may have been useful in this case.*

FURTHER READING

Brimacombe J, Berry A. A review of anaesthesia for ruptured abdominal aortic aneurysm with special emphasis on preclamping fluid resuscitation. Anaesth Intensive Care 1993; 21: 311–323

Crawford E S. Ruptured abdominal aortic aneurysm: an editorial. Vascular Surg 1991; 13: 348–350

Nolan J P. Techniques for rapid fluid infusion. Br J Intensive Care 1993; 98–105

Amighi D A, Farnell I V, Mucha P, Listrup D M, Anderson D L. Prospective randomised trial of rapid venous access for patients in hypovolaemic shock. Ann Emerg Med 1989; 18: 927–930

Murphy W G, Davies M J, Eduardo B J. The haemostatic response to surgery and trauma. Br J Anaes 1993; 70(2): 205–213

Kulka P J, Tryba M. Inotropic support of the critically ill patient. Drugs 1993; 45: 654–667

4 Porphyria

A 21-year-old 55 kg female was admitted to the on call surgical unit with abdominal pain of 48 hours duration. The pain was colicky in nature and appeared more prominent in the lower-right quadrant of her abdomen. During the preceding 12 hours she had vomited at regular intervals. On examination she appeared unwell, anxious, emotionally labile and dehydrated. Her temperature was recorded as 38°C, heart rate 150/min and blood pressure 170/110 mmHg. Further questioning about her symptoms revealed she had experienced similar abdominal pains intermittently during the previous 3 years mainly related to menstruation, but the intensity and duration of the pains had increased. In addition to the abdominal pain she complained of weakness of her upper arms and shoulders. She had recently commenced treatment with the oral contraceptive pill. Investigations revealed a haemoglobin of 140 g/l with an elevated haematocrit of 0.51, WBC $13.2 \times 10^{-9}/l$. Urea was mildly elevated at 8.4 mmol/l with a creatinine of 119 mmol/l. Electrolyte analysis revealed serum sodium 128 mmol/l and chloride 96 mmol/l. Abdominal and chest X-rays were within normal limits.

A diagnosis of acute appendicitis was assumed. Initial fluid resuscitation was commenced with 0.9% sodium chloride, but she became more restless and at times confused. The surgical team decided that a laparotomy should be undertaken with the minimum of delay. She was taken to theatre and anaesthetised with a rapid sequence induction using thiopentone and suxamethonium. Thereafter anaesthesia was maintained with enflurane and nitrous oxide in oxygen, with morphine for analgesia and atracurium for muscle relaxation. Throughout the course of the operation the blood pressure remained at pre-anaesthetic values and the tachycardia persisted.

At operation the appendix was not inflamed and limited examination of the pelvis revealed no acute pathology. Muscle relaxation was antagonised with neostigmine, but in view of the tachycardia no anticholinergic agent was administered. The patient was very slow to recover spontaneous respiration and consciousness, and when she did so was acutely confused. She was admitted to a high-dependency unit following recovery. Her condition deteriorated with progressive hypertension, tachycardia and hypoxaemia and she was transferred to the Intensive Therapy Unit.

DISCUSSION POINTS

The history and examination described here is reasonably detailed and there are a number of points that suggest further exploration and investigation might reveal a different diagnosis. The examination findings are characteristic of a patient with an acute attack of porphyria.

- *Question 1:* *Which features in the history and examination would lead you to this conclusion?*

Acute intermittent porphyria is a rare but important condition for the anaesthetist as many anaesthetic drugs are porphyrinogenic. The porphyrias are classified into hepatic and erythropoietic, acute and non-acute. It is only the hepatic acute porphyrias – acute intermittent porphyria (AIP), variegate porphyria (VP), hereditary coproporphyria (HC) – that are of importance to the anaesthetist. The synthesis of haem from its precursors glycine and succinyl CoA involves a series of enzymatic reactions first creating aminolaevulinic acid (ALA), then the monopyrrole porphobilinogen (PBG), isomerising them into a tetra-pyrrole ring, finally chelating with iron to form haem. Depletion of enzymes (uroporphyrinogen I synthase-AIP, protoporphyrinogen oxidase-VP, coproporphyrinogen oxidase-HC) causes an increase in certain porphyrins detected in the urine. All patients with an attack of porphyria excrete ALA and PBG in excess in their urine. Diagnostic urine testing is with Ehrlich's aldehyde, urine turning a pink red colour with its addition.

Most drugs that are porphyrinogenic stimulate the enzyme dALA synthase increasing ALA and are generally inducers of the P450 enzyme system. Conflicting data exists regarding anaesthetic drugs which are safe to use in patients with porphyria.

- *Question 2:* *Which drugs appear safe to use?*

● **Question 3:** *Was the anaesthetic technique used in this case appropriate?*

● **Question 4:** *What problems should be anticipated in a patient with an acute attack of porphyria, and how should such a patient be managed?*

FURTHER READING

Harrison G C, Meissner P N, Hift R J. Anaesthesia for the porphyric patient (review). Anaesthesia 1993; 48: 417–421
Harrison J C, McAuley F T. Propofol for sedation in intensive care in a patient with an acute porphyric attack. Anaesthesia 1992; 47: 355–6

5 Amitriptyline overdose

The anaesthetic registrar was called to the Accident and Emergency Department (A&E) to assist in the management of a 16-year-old girl believed to have swallowed 50 of her mother's amitriptyline tablets following an argument with her boyfriend. She was brought to A&E by her parents who found her in a drowsy and confused condition. She became unrousable shortly before arrival at hospital. Her parents reported that she had no significant past medical history and was on no medication.

On arrival in A&E, her respiration was noted to be shallow and Glasgow Coma Scale (GCS) was 7. Her pupils were widely dilated but reactive and there was no gag reflex. On establishing ECG and non-invasive blood pressure monitoring, a broad-complex tachycardia (rate 160/min) and blood pressure of 160/110 mmHg were revealed. Twelve lead ECG showed the QRS interval to be greater than 0.12 s. In order to protect the airway and permit gastric lavage, endotracheal intubation was performed. This was accomplished easily without neuromuscular blockade. Ventilation was assisted and there was only minimal return of tablets on gastric lavage. Fifty grams of activated charcoal were instilled into the stomach after the washout and arrangements made for transfer to the intensive care unit. Serum electrolytes, full blood count and arterial blood gases were all within normal limits. On arrival in the intensive care unit, some 15 minutes later, blood pressure had fallen to 85/60 mmHg but peripheral perfusion remained good. A radial arterial line was established, but as this was being connected to the transducer her heart rate increased to 180/min and blood pressure fell to 40 mmHg systolic. When carotid sinus massage failed to control the tachycardia, metoprolol was given which slowed the heart rate to 140/min and the blood pressure rose to 90/60 mmHg.

Ten minutes later she had a grand mal seizure, followed immediately by ventricular fibrillation. External cardiac compression was commenced, and FiO_2 increased to 1.0 as the defibrillator was charged. A prolonged period of resuscitation followed during which she received multiple shocks, at first 200 and then 360 joules and intravenous adrenaline according to Resuscitation Council guidelines. Sodium bicarbonate was given after each 15 minutes of resuscitation time. She had several further seizures for which she received diazemuls and then phenytoin and thiopentone. After 60 minutes sinus rhythm was established and her condition stabilised with a tachycardia of 140/min and blood pressure of 100/50 mmHg. At this time mannitol was given in an attempt to minimise cerebral oedema. Ventilation was continued overnight, maintaining a $PaCO_2$ between 3.5 and 4.0 kPa. It was possible to reduce the FiO_2 to 0.4 while maintaining a PaO_2 above 13 kPa. Over the next 12 hours there were signs of a lightening level of consciousness and morphine and midazolam were given to provide sedation. Ventilation was continued for 24 hours. The next day, when the sedation was withdrawn, she woke and responded appropriately to commands. She was extubated, and following a further 24 hours invasive monitoring in the intensive care unit was transferred to the medical ward. There was no evidence of neurological impairment. Four days later she was discharged from hospital after psychiatric counselling. The psychiatric assessment did not demonstrate evidence of any suicidal intent.

DISCUSSION POINTS

Self-poisoning accounts for 95% of all poisoning-related admissions, and is one of the most common causes of non-traumatic coma in the young. Para-suicide (i.e. deliberate, often impulsive self-poisoning without suicidal intent) is more common in young women than men, and often occurs in response to a 'crisis' event, such as in this case. Management of most poisoning consists of general supportive measures, however, there are more specific measures required for some drugs (e.g. acetylcysteine and paracetamol poisoning).

● *Question 1: Discuss how you would assess and manage a patient following a suspected self-poisoning. What general measures would you take? Discuss ways to increase drug elimination from the body.*

Amitriptyline is an important cause of death from poisoning. More than 15 mg/kg may be fatal.

● *Question 2: What typical signs and symptoms would you expect to see?*

If cardiac arrest occurs, cardiac massage may have to be continued for prolonged periods. Cardiac bypass has been used in several cases to support the circulation.

Antidysrhythmics, especially membrane-stabilising drugs, should be avoided in this group of patients, although phenytoin, dopamine and dobutamine are probably safe.

- *Question 3:* Why is this?

- *Question 4:* Discuss the effect of pH elevation on elimination of amitriptyline.

- *Question 5:* Describe the European Resuscitation Council guidelines for the management of ventricular fibrillation, asystole and electromechanical dissociation.

FURTHER READING

College G G, Hanson G C. The management of acute poisoning. Br J Anaes 1993; 70: 562–573

Frommer D, Kulig K, Marx J, Rumack B. Tricyclic antidepressant overdose: a review. JAMA 1987; 257: 521–6

Goodwin D A, Lally K P, Null D M. Extracorporeal membrane oxygenation support for cardiac dysfunction from tricyclic antidepressant overdose. Critical Care Med 1993; 21: 625

Levitt M, Sullivan J, Owens S, Burnham L, Finlay P. Amitriptyline plasma protein binding: effect of plasma pH and relevance to clinical overdose. Am J Emerg Med 1986; 4: 121–125

European Resuscitation Council Working Party. Adult advanced cardiac life support: the European Resuscitation Council guidelines 1992 (abridged). BMJ 1993; 306: 1589–93

6 TURP syndrome

A 76-year-old man was scheduled to undergo elective transurethral resection of prostate (TURP) for benign prostatic hypertrophy.

Pre-operative assessment revealed long-standing severe chronic obstructive pulmonary disease (COPD) with an exercise tolerance of approximately 200 yards. In addition, within the past three months he had experienced several episodes of central chest pain, characteristic of angina pectoris. On examination he was plethoric with a hyperinflated chest. Auscultation revealed scattered rhonchi and basal crepitations which cleared with coughing. Blood pressure was recorded at 160/90 mmHg and a regular pulse rate of 82/min. Current medication included terbutaline, ipratropium and budesonide inhalers together with enteric coated prednisolone tablets, isosorbide mononitrate and GTN sublingual spray as required.

Investigations included a chest X-ray which showed the classic features of COPD and a small area of right-sided basal collapse. ECG showed sinus rhythm, left bundle branch block, Q-waves in leads II and III, and inverted T-waves in the lateral chest leads. Haematological results were as follows: haemoglobin 168 g/l, platelets 430, WCC 14.9×10^9l. Arterial blood gases on air showed: PaO_2 9.8 kPa; $PaCO_2$ 7.3 kPa; pH 7.48; HCO_3 29 mmol/l; and base excess of +5. Urea and electrolytes were within normal limits.

After consultation with the patient, the operation was performed under spinal anaesthesia which was achieved with the intrathecal injection of plain bupivacaine. Supplementary oxygen 6L/min was given via a Hudson mask, and over the course of the following six minutes the blood pressure fell from 165/90 mmHg to 75/40 mmHg. The patient complained of chest pain which was relieved with the restoration of the blood pressure with increments of ephedrine, together with rapid intravenous infusion of 500 ml of crystalloid solution. Midazolam was then given intravenously for sedation and surgery commenced. Twenty-five minutes into the resection the surgeon commented that there appeared to be excessive bleeding from the prostatic bed and asked for the recorded blood pressure. It was measured as 146/78 mmHg. After a further 12 minutes the SpO_2 was noted to fall from 97% to 91% and the blood pressure to rise to 200/90 mmHg. The patient became restless and agitated.

TURP syndrome was suspected and the surgeon was asked to terminate the procedure. The patient was transferred to the recovery room. On arrival he complained of breathlessness and diminished vision. As blood was being taken the patient appeared to have a grand mal seizure. He became apnoeic and ventricular fibrillation was seen on the ECG monitor. Cardiopulmonary resuscitation ensued with restoration of sinus rhythm and cardiac output. Respiratory effort remained poor and the patient was ventilated and transferred to the intensive care unit for further management.

On admission chest X-ray revealed gross pulmonary oedema and a 12-lead ECG showed signs of an acute inferior myocardial infarction.

DISCUSSION POINTS

For patients with respiratory disease, spinal anaesthesia is considered to have some advantages over general anaesthesia for prostatic surgery.

- *Question 1:* *In view of this patient's past medical history and subsequent TURP syndrome, critically comment on the pre-anaesthetic assessment and choice of anaesthetic technique used in this case.*

- *Question 2:* *Discuss the presentation, treatment and prophylaxis of the TURP syndrome with particular reference to the issue of fluid replacement and the restoration of normal biochemical values.*

Transient blindness is occasionally a feature of the TURP syndrome. Several reasons have been suggested for this including the use of glycine 1.5% as the intra-operative irrigating fluid.

- *Question 3:* *Discuss the evidence for this together with the nature and metabolism of glycine.*

FURTHER READING

Hatch P D. Surgical and anaesthetic considerations in the transurethral resection of prostate. (review). Anaes and Intensive Care 1987; 15: 203–11

Jensen V. The TURP syndrome. Can J Anaes 1991; 38: 90–7

Mackenzie A R. Influence of anaesthesia on blood loss in transurethral prostatectomy. Scottish Med J 1990; 35: 14–16

7 Recent myocardial infarction

A 67-year-old woman presented to the gynaecologists with post-menopausal bleeding. Although she had suffered from angina pectoris for five years her symptoms were well controlled. Current medication consisted of atenolol and aspirin. Six weeks previously she had been admitted and treated for an anterior myocardial infarction from which she had made an uneventful recovery. She was scheduled for a dilatation and curettage under general anaesthesia but after further deliberation it was thought wiser to attempt an endometrial biopsy in view of the recent myocardial infarction. This procedure was carried out successfully and revealed an endometrial carcinoma. The treatment of choice was abdominal hysterectomy, but it was felt that surgery could safely be deferred until three months after the myocardial infarction.

On admission for hysterectomy she did not complain of any symptoms relating to myocardial ischaemia. Medication was unchanged and history and examination were unremarkable with a heart rate of 55/min and a blood pressure of 150/80 mmHg. In particular, there was no evidence of cardiac failure and all investigations were normal apart from ECG changes consistent with a previous myocardial infarction. A cardiology opinion was sought and it was agreed that since no invasive management of her heart condition was envisaged, no further investigation was warranted.

Atenolol and lorazepam were given orally two hours prior to anaesthesia, and thereafter oxygen was given by face mask in the ward and during transport to the anaesthetic room. Peripheral venous access was established, and following further sedation with intravenous midazolam, a radial arterial line and a pulmonary artery catheter were inserted under local anaesthesia. An epidural catheter was introduced via a Tuohy needle in the L3/4 interspace and bupivacaine was injected in increments until the upper level of block to pinprick was at T6. During establishment of the block intravenous fluids were given to maintain the systolic blood pressure above 100 mmHg. The pulmonary capillary wedge pressure was also monitored and remained less than 10 mmHg. The ST segments of the ECG leads I, II and V2 were monitored and the trends recorded. General anaesthesia was induced with droperidol, alfentanil and etomidate and muscle relaxation achieved with vecuronium. During laryngoscopy and intubation the heart rate increased from 55/min to 68/min and the systolic blood pressure from 100 mmHg to 120 mmHg, but there were no ECG changes suggestive of myocardial ischaemia. Anaesthesia was maintained with enflurane and nitrous oxide in oxygen, and surgery proceeded. Shortly after surgery commenced ST segment depression (about 0.8 mm) was noted. This persisted for two minutes and was successfully treated with intravenous glyceryl trinitrate but otherwise all recordings remained stable throughout the operation.

After surgery she was extubated and transferred, breathing spontaneously and pain-free, to the intensive care unit. Postoperative analgesia was achieved with an epidural infusion of 0.1% bupivacaine for the first 24 hours followed by intravenous morphine via a patient controlled analgesia system. Thereafter her recovery was uneventful.

DISCUSSION POINTS

One study has demonstrated a re-infarction rate of 27% in patients undergoing non-cardiac surgery within 3 months of a myocardial infarction and 11% if the infarct had occurred 4–6 months previously.

● *Question 1: How convincing is the evidence that invasive monitoring and aggressive therapy with intravenous fluids and vaso-active drugs can reduce this incidence?*

● *Question 2: What therapy would you use if you suspected ischaemia from the ECG?*

Transoesophageal echocardiography is a sensitive method of detecting changes in ventricular wall motion which may be associated with myocardial ischaemia.

- *Question 3:* Was the monitoring of this patient adequate, or should this further technique been used?

- *Question 4:* Was the cardiological assessment adequate prior to this operation?

- *Question 5:* In what circumstances would you recommend assessment of ejection fraction prior to anaesthesia and surgery?

There are numerous methods for pre-treating patients to try to avoid the tachycardia and hypertension associated with laryngoscopy and intubation.

- *Question 6:* What would you have recommended in this patient?

Myocardial ischaemia has commonly been detected some days after surgery.

- *Question 7:* *Was this patient fully monitored long enough to confirm that this did not occur?*

FURTHER READING

Fleisher L A, Barash P G. Preoperative cardiac evaluation for non-cardiac surgery. A functional approach. Anes Analg (1992) 74: 586–598

Goldman L, Caldera D L, Nussbaum S R, Southwick F S, Krogstad D, Murray B, Burke D S et al. Multifactorial index of cardiac risk in non-cardiac surgical procedures. New Eng J Med 1977; 297: 845–850

Steen P A, Tinker J H, Tarhan S. Myocardial re-infarction after anesthesia and surgery. JAMA 1978; 239: 2566–2570

Rao T L K, Jacobs K H, El-Etr A A. Reinfarction following anaesthesia in patients with myocardial infarction. Anesthesiology 1983; 59: 499–505

Lowenstein E, Yusuf S, Teplick R S. Perioperative myocardial reinfarction: a glimmer of hope – a note of caution. Anesthesiology 1983; 59: 493–494

Edwards N D, Reilly C S. Detection of peri-operative myocardial ischaemia. Br J Anaes 1994; 72: 104–115

8 Ankylosing spondylitis

A 58-year-old 75 kg man was admitted as an emergency with a history of acute upper abdominal pain. He suffered from long-standing ankylosing spondylitis, and current medication consisted of indomethacin and ranitidine. Past medical history included prostatitis and recent investigation of breathlessness. He had had no previous anaesthetics. On admission he was conscious but pale and sweating. Examination of the abdomen revealed generalised tenderness and rebound tenderness. His arterial blood pressure was 90/55 mmHg and the heart rate 115/min. Two large intravenous cannulae were sited and fluid resuscitation commenced. Blood was taken for routine haematology, urea and electrolytes and cross-match. Within 40 minutes the haemodynamic parameters had stabilised and emergency laparotomy was proposed.

Assessment by the anaesthetist revealed a completely ankylosed spine with severe kyphosis of the cervical region and a rigid thoracic cage. Temporo-mandibular involvement limited jaw opening to 2 cm. The patient had a full set of teeth. A portable chest X-ray showed bilateral upper lobe fibrosis with several large cysts and an enlarged heart. An abdominal film revealed marked ankylosis of the spine (Fig. 8.1). An ECG showed

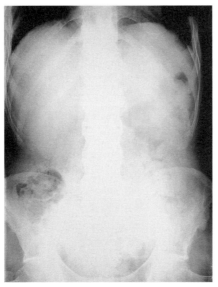

Fig. 8.1 Abdominal X-ray showing ankylosis

left ventricular hypertrophy. Chest auscultation revealed an early blowing diastolic murmur at the left sternal edge and a systolic flow murmur. Conventional rapid sequence induction was thought to be impossible due to the degree of mouth opening and extent of neck flexion. It was felt that tracheostomy under local anaesthetic would prove difficult because of the neck deformity.

Awake nasal fibre optic intubation in the sitting position was undertaken. Local anaesthetic spray was applied to the nasal mucosa and to provide oral and pharyngeal anaesthesia. The superior laryngeal nerves were blocked using pledgets soaked in 4% lignocaine positioned in the pyriform fossae using Krauss's forceps. The inferior aspect of the larynx and trachea were anaesthetised with 4% lignocaine applied by crico-thyroid puncture. After placing graded nasal pharyngeal airways coated in lignocaine gel in the nostril, a nasal endotracheal tube was placed through the right nostril. This was then advanced into the trachea with the use of a paediatric fibre-optic bronchoscope. Having secured the airway, general anaesthesia was induced with etomidate and maintained with isoflurane and 70% nitrous oxide in oxygen. Neuromuscular blockade and analgesia were obtained with atracurium and morphine.

Laparotomy revealed a perforated duodenal ulcer which was over-sewn, and vagotomy and pyloroplasty were performed. At the conclusion of the procedure the patient was transferred to the Intensive Care Unit for ventilation. The following morning after careful assessment of respiratory function, the patient was extubated and further recovery was uneventful.

DISCUSSION POINTS

In addition to their skeletal deformities, patients with ankylosing spondylitis have a number of other extra-articular conditions.

- *Question 1:* *Discuss the cardiovascular, pulmonary and neurological manifestations of this disease that may concern an anaesthetist.*

Cervical fracture is common in patients with ankylosing spondylitis, often leading to quadriplegia. Airway management in patients who have long-standing ankylosing spondylitis is of the utmost concern to the anaesthetist. Part of this management will necessarily involve manipulation of the cervical spine.

• **Question 2:** *Outline the various manoeuvres and techniques available to aid airway control and intubation in these patients while at the same time minimising the risk of trauma to the cervical spine.*

Patients with ankylosing spondylitis commonly present for orthopaedic procedures, including total hip replacement.

• **Question 3:** *Discuss anaesthetic techniques suitable for such operations.*

Fibre-optic laryngoscopy requires skill and familiarity with the technique to accomplish the procedure with safety and minimal distress to the patient. Local anaesthesia of the upper airway will increase the chance of aspiration should the patient vomit or regurgitate. In a case such as this, however, this risk can hardly be avoided without exposing the patient to even greater hazards.

FURTHER READING

Sinclair J R, Mason R A. Ankylosing spondylitis (the case for awake intubation). Anaesthesia 1984; 39: 3–11
Salathe M, Johr M. Unsuspected cervical fractures: a common problem with ankylosing spondilitis. Anesthesiology 1989; 70: 869–70
Cobley M, Vaughan R S. Recognition and management of difficult airway problems (review). Br J Anaes 1992; 68: 90–7
Vaughan R S. Teaching fibre optic laryngoscopy. Br J Anaes 1991; 66: 538–40
Haslock I. Ankylosing spondylitis (review of the respiratory aspects of ankylosing spondylitis). Balliere's Clinical Rheumatology 1993; 7: 99–115
O'Neill T W, Bresnihan B. The heart in ankylosing spondylitis. Ann Rheum Dis 1992; 51: 705–6

9 Drug abuse

An 18-year-old male was admitted to the Accident and Emergency (A&E) department after being found unconscious at home by his girlfriend. No history was obtainable from the patient, but his girlfriend reported he had complained of a 'flu like' illness over the past week, with aching joints and low back pain. He had experienced severe shivering attacks and night sweats. The day before he had complained of a headache and had vomited on several occasions. Paramedic staff reported a self-limiting right-sided focal seizure en route to hospital.

On admission the patient had a Glasgow coma score of 10, appeared cachectic and multiple injection marks were found on his arms, hands and groin. In addition there was a left groin abscess measuring 3 cm × 4 cm. On further questioning the girlfriend admitted they both abused intravenous drugs and shared needles. She thought her boyfriend had had hepatitis in the past, but had refused an HIV test. However, she volunteered that she had tested positive for the HIV virus.

Further examination of the patient revealed central cyanosis, vasculitic skin lesions with areas of haemorrhagic necrosis and multiple splinter haemorrhages. He was in atrial fibrillation with a ventricular rate of 150/min, blood pressure was 90/50 mmHg and the respiratory rate 28/min. Although he felt cold peripherally, rectal temperature was recorded as 38.5°C. Chest auscultation revealed a pan systolic murmur grade 2/6, radiating to the axilla, and widespread fine crepitations in both lung fields. Examination of the neck revealed giant 'v' waves, suggestive of tricuspid incompetence. Arterial blood gases on air showed hypoxaemia with moderate respiratory alkalosis (Table 1). Changes consistent with pulmonary oedema were evident on the chest X-ray (Fig. 9.1).

Table 1 Blood results on admission

pH	7.51
$PaCO_2$	3.2 kPa
PaO_2	6.3 kPa
st bic	26 mmol/l
base excess	+3
urea	37.5 mmol/l
creatinine	430 mmol/l
Hb	97 g/l
WCC	23×10^9/l

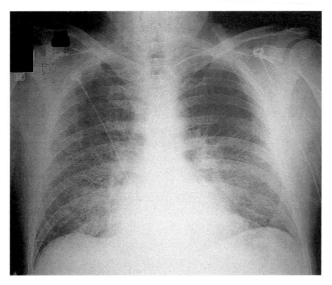

Fig. 9.1 Chest X-ray showing changes consistent with bilateral pulmonary oedema

On the basis of his history and these findings a diagnosis of subacute bacterial endocarditis was made. A CT scan of the head was ordered prior to transfer to the intensive care unit. The patient was intubated in the emergency room following pre-oxygenation and the administration of thiopentone and suxamethonium. Intermittent positive pressure ventilation was undertaken with an oxygen and air mixture (FiO_2 0.5) and anaesthesia maintained with a propofol infusion. CT revealed a lesion consistent with a left-sided parieto-temporal abscess. Blood results revealed acute renal failure and a normochromic normocytic anaemia and leukocytosis (Table 1). Following a short period of stabilisation and insertion of invasive monitoring in the Intensive Care Unit, the patient underwent burr hole drainage of the cerebral abscess and incision and drainage of the groin abscess.

On return to the intensive care unit transoesophageal echocardiography was performed revealing severe mitral valve incompetence with vegetations. His condition deteriorated in the next 24 hours, with increasing cardiovascular instability and worsening pulmonary oedema. It was decided to proceed to emergency mitral valve replacement. Following successful surgery he spent a further 13 days in the intensive care unit and required haemodialysis. Weaning from ventilatory support was prolonged and during this time he displayed labile blood pressure, sweats, tachycardia and was agitated.

A full recovery was eventually made and he was referred to a drug rehabilitation unit for further assistance with his drug addiction.

DISCUSSION POINTS

Substance abusers are frequent attendees at A&E, presenting with a variety of conditions. In this case the presentation was of endocarditis.

● *Question 1:* *Suggest other medical and surgical problems associated with habitual substance abuse.*

In the absence of a clinical history, the patient with reduced level of consciousness presents a diagnostic challenge.

● *Question 2:* *What features in the presentation and examination might lead you to suspect substance abuse?*

It is important to remember substance-abusing patients abuse multiple drugs, and a high degree of suspicion is necessary to determine other compounds the patient is taking e.g., alcohol, heroin or cocaine. Cocaine abuse has increased in this country during the last decade. Free base cocaine is a pure cocaine alkaloid produced by ether extraction and 'crack' is made by heating cocaine hydrochloride with baking soda or ammonia, resulting in a precipitate which is smokeable and contains adulterants.

● *Question 3:* *Outline the effects cocaine substance abuse may have on the cardiovascular and pulmonary systems.*

Intravenous substance abusers have a significant risk of both hepatitis infection and HIV infection. This poses a potential infective risk for all staff treating these patients.

• **Question 4:** *Discuss which measures should be adopted to reduce this risk to personnel in the operating room and intensive care unit.*

• **Question 5:** *In the event of contamination of a member of staff with blood from an HIV infected individual, is there still a place for the prophylactic use of zidovudine (AZT)?*

Substance-abusers requiring elective or emergency surgery pose a number of problems for the anaesthetist for premedication, anaesthetic technique and pain relief.

• **Question 6:** *Discuss these problems and how you might manage them.*

A substance-abuser, whether addicted to opiates, benzodiazepines, alcohol or other substances, if denied access to his or her routine supply, may develop withdrawal features.

● **Question 7:** *Describe some of these features related to the drugs mentioned above and how you might manage the patient.*

● **Question 8:** *What other problems might the alcohol-abusing patient have in the perioperative period?*

FURTHER READING

Wood P R, Soni N. Anaesthesia and substance abuse. Anaesthesia 1989; 44: 672–80
Jeffries D J. HIV and hepatitis – some way to go (editorial). Anaesthesia 1992; 47: 921–22
AIDS and hepatitis B. Guidelines for anaesthetists. London: Association for Anaesthetists, 1988
Jeffries D J. Zidovudine after occupational exposure to HIV. BMJ 1991; 302: 1349–51
Tonnesen H, Petersen K, Hojgaard L, Stokholm K H, Nielsen H J, Knigge U, Kehlet H. Postoperative morbidity among symptom-free alcohol misusers. Lancet 1992; 340: 334–7
Brody S L, Slovis C M, Wrenn K D. Cocaine-related medical problems: consecutive series of 233 patients. Am J Med 1990; 88: 325–331

10

Hypoxaemia during hip arthroplasty

A 76-year-old male presented for right total hip replacement. Past medical history consisted of osteoarthritis and long-standing chronic obstructive airways disease which was treated with inhaled steroids and a β_2 adrenergic agonist. He admitted to breathlessness on exertion, although the severity of this was difficult to assess due to exercise limitation from hip pain. Physical examination was unremarkable other than diffuse rhonchi on chest auscultation. Chest X-ray was characteristic of emphysema, and there was some lateral ischaemia on the ECG. Pulmonary function tests revealed a FEVL of 600 ml and a FVC of 2500 ml. Peak expiratory flow rate was 100 L/min, and there was little reversibility with bronchodilators. Other investigations were unremarkable.

He was premedicated with temazepam orally one hour prior to anaesthesia. After establishing venous access and basic monitoring the patient was turned to the left lateral position and a 25G Whitacre needle was inserted to the sub-arachnoid space at the third lumbar intervertebral space. Spinal anaesthesia was established with the injection of hyperbaric bupivacaine. He was then turned supine and after 15 minutes the upper level of analgesia reached T6. During this time he received 500 ml of gelatin solution and oxygen 4 L/min via a Hudson mask. The blood pressure dropped from 160/90 mmHg to 120/70 mmHg.

He was repositioned into the left lateral position for surgery and a propofol infusion was commenced to provide sedation. An additional small bolus of propofol was given as surgery commenced. He remained stable and slept peacefully for the initial 30 minutes of surgery. It was then noted the oxygen saturation fell from 99% to 76% over about 30 seconds. All other parameters remained stable and ventilation appeared adequate. Whilst surgery continued, the propofol infusion was discontinued and after checking that there was no evidence of gastric contents in the pharynx, the lungs were manually inflated with 100% oxygen via a face mask and Bain-type breathing system. The oxygen saturation rose to 85–90%, and after about one minute the patient awoke. Due to the patient's position, physical examination of the chest was difficult, but it appeared that there was decreased air entry at the left apex. He was comfortable and complained of no symptoms, so high-flow oxygen continued via the face mask and he was encouraged to breath deeply and cough. The oxygen saturation remained at 85–90% until surgery was completed.

On turning the patient supine the signs of left upper lobe collapse were evident, with poor expansion, dullness to percussion and no air entry in

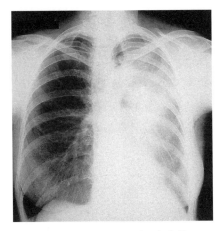

Fig. 10.1 Chest X-ray showing Left Upper Lobe collapse

that area. This diagnosis was confirmed with chest X-ray (Fig. 10.1). He was treated with good effect by intensive chest physiotherapy and postural drainage in the recovery room. Within 30 minutes the oxygen saturation had again risen to 99%. Lung re-expansion was confirmed by chest X-ray.

DISCUSSION POINTS

Pulse oximetry played an important role in the safety of this patient.

● *Question 1: Describe the signs which might have led you to suspect intra-operative hypoxaemia if this monitoring had not been available.*

● *Question 2: Intravenous sedation may depress the cough reflex. Discuss whether another technique would have been more appropriate in this patient.*

Adverse reactions may occur during joint surgery and procedures involving the use of cement have particularly been implicated.

● **Question 3:** *What would you expect to see during these reactions, what are possible mechanisms of these reactions and how can they be minimised?*

This patient's hypoxaemia responded well to simple measures.

● **Question 4:** *What treatment options would be open to you if severe hypoxaemia had persisted?*

● **Question 5:** *Discuss the differential diagnosis of intra-operative hypoxaemia in this patient.*

FURTHER READING

Association of Anaesthetists of Great Britain and Ireland. Recommendations for standards of monitoring during anaesthesia and recovery. Report of a Working Party, July 1988

Nolan J P. Arterial oxygenation and mean arterial blood pressure in patients undergoing total hip replacement: cemented versus uncemented components. Anaesthesia 1994; 49: 293–299

Al-Shaikh B. Effect of inspired oxygen concentrations in the incidence of desaturation in patients undergoing total hip replacement. Br J Anaes 1991; 66: 580–582

11

Free flap transfer

A 40-year-old woman who had previously undergone a right mastectomy was scheduled for a free flap transfer for the purpose for reconstructing her breast. She was otherwise in good health. On the evening preceding and the day of surgery she received temazepam. Induction of anaesthesia was standard and maintained with isoflurane in oxygen and nitrous oxide. A large-bore venous and a radial arterial cannula were sited. Her arms and head were covered, but the nature of the surgery precluded covering abdomen and chest. Her legs were covered with a warm air mattress. Intravenous fluid was warmed and inspired gases were administered via a circle system with a heat and moisture exchange filter at the patient end of the system.

The surgery lasted 6 hours during which time fluid input, urine output and blood loss were measured. Prior to the microvascular anastomosis, an infusion of glyceryl trinitrate was commenced but blood pressure was maintained. After removing the vascular clips the perfusion of the flap did not look adequate. Following a bolus dose of glycopyrrolate which increased the heart rate from 60 to 90/min, perfusion of the flap was seen to improve. When surgery was completed the patient was transferred to the recovery room where her temperature measured via the nasopharynx was 36°C. A brief period of shivering resolved spontaneously and she was returned to the ward for specialist nursing in a warmed room.

DISCUSSION POINTS

Free flap transfers using microvascular techniques are common procedures in plastic and reconstructive surgery and the anaesthetist has an important role to play in the successful outcome. Adequate tissue perfusion must be maintained and it is important to keep the blood pressure near normal and to reduce peripheral vascular resistance.

- *Question 1: What drugs can be employed and what drugs should be avoided?*

Temperature control is important during prolonged surgery.

- *Question 2:* *Why does the temperature drop during anaesthesia?*

- *Question 3:* *What sites in the body are available for temperature sensing and how accurate are these measurements?*

- *Question 4:* *Is postoperative shivering purely related to a reduction in body temperature?*

Some authorities feel that it is important to maintain plasma osmotic pressure by infusing warmed colloid solutions to replace even modest blood loss.

- *Question 5:* *What are the fluid requirements during this type of surgery and how may they be estimated and maintained in an otherwise fit patient?*

● **Question 6:** *Is it necessary to monitor central venous pressure in this case?*

In order to reduce heat and moisture loss from the respiratory tract, a circle system and heat and moisture exchanger were used in conjunction in this instance.

● **Question 7:** *Describe how this would benefit the patient.*

● **Question 8:** *Outline the various methods available for humidification of inspired gases and their relative effectiveness.*

● **Question 9:** *What other methods are available to minimise temperature change during anaesthesia, and what are the practical problems associated with these methods?*

Regional anaesthesia produces sympathetic block and vasodilation and is popular in some centres. However, the transplanted vessels are already denervated and the use of a local anaesthetic technique does not diminish the need for attention to the other factors above.

FURTHER READING

Macdonald D J F. Anaesthesia for microvascular surgery: a physiological approach.
  Br J Anaes 1985; 57: 904–912
Imrie M M, Hall G M. Body temperature and anaesthesia. Br J Anaes 1990; 64: 306–314
Simpson P. Peri-operative blood loss and its reduction: the role of the anaesthetist.
  Br J Anaes 1992; 69: 498–507
Hedley R M, Allt-Graham J. Heat and moisture exchangers and breathing filters. Br J Anaes
  1994; 73: 227–236

12 Post operative nausea and vomiting

A 22-year-old woman was admitted at 11.30 am as a day-case for elective removal of wisdom teeth. She lived alone in student accommodation but had arranged for a friend to stay overnight after her discharge from hospital. Systematic enquiry, physical examination and urinalysis did not reveal any findings of note and no further investigations were performed. No premedication was given and she was taken to theatre at 2 p.m. She was first seen by the anaesthetist in the anaesthetic room. Basic monitoring was established, intravenous access obtained and anaesthesia was induced with propofol and fentanyl. Mivacurium was administered and intubation with a cuffed nasal endotracheal tube accomplished without difficulty. Anaesthesia was maintained with isoflurane in nitrous oxide and oxygen with intermittent positive pressure ventilation, and a throat pack was inserted. At the completion of surgery some ten minutes later neostigmine and glycopyrrolate were administered and the throat pack removed.

In the recovery room she complained of pain and morphine was administered intravenously in increments. Her pain settled but she then complained of nausea. Metoclopramide was administered but had no effect. She continued to complain of nausea particularly when sitting up and was unable to get out of bed. She tried to take sips of water but this induced vomiting blood-stained fluid. Ondansetron was then administered and this led to a rapid resolution of her symptoms. The development of postoperative nausea and vomiting meant that she was not fit for discharge home by the closure time of the day-bed unit and she required transfer to an inpatient facility.

DISCUSSION POINTS

This patient was first seen and assessed by the anaesthetist in the anaesthetic room. It may have been impractical to make any other arrangement but this is clearly less than ideal.

- *Question 1: Describe the facilities you would incorporate if you were designing a new day-case unit, giving consideration to patient assessment and recovery, staffing and timing of operating lists.*

- *Question 2:* Is it acceptable to undertake day-case surgery on an afternoon list – especially if the day ward is not available in the early evening?

- *Question 3:* Postoperative pain relief is important in this situation. Do you think it wise to administer an opioid to a patient who will be discharged some hours later?

- *Question 4:* What are the important factors which predispose to the occurrence of postoperative nausea and vomiting?

- *Question 5:* What criteria would you use to decide when to employ prophylactic drug therapy for the prevention of nausea and vomiting?

- *Question 6:* If an anti-emetic is to be given prophyllactically, when should this be done – at the start of anaesthesia, or at the end?

Fasting patients prior to elective surgery, often for at least 6 hours, has long been advocated to reduce the stomach contents and hence the risk of aspiration.

- *Question 7:* *Are there disadvantages to this policy?*

- *Question 8:* *Could a shorter fasting period be more advantageous for the patient?*

- *Question 9:* *Is the incidence of postoperative nausea and vomiting related to this?*

The use of local anaesthetic agents can dramatically reduce the need for opiates if time, care and attention to detail are taken. This is not possible for all operative sites but is an underused technique which has much to offer. Many would consider this to be particularly relevant for a case involving a patient with a known history of emesis.

FURTHER READING

Royal College of Surgeons of England. Commission on the provision of surgical services: Guidelines for day-case surgery. July 1985

Goodwin A P L, Ogg T W. Pre-operative preparation for day surgery. BMJ 1992; 47: 197–201.

Russell D, Kenny G N C. 5-HT3 antagonists in postoperative nausea and vomiting. Br J Anaes 1992; 69 (suppl 1): 63S–68S

Haigh C G, Kaplan L A, Durham J M, Dupeyron J P, Harmer M, Kenny G N C. Nausea and
    vomiting after gynaecological surgery: a meta-analysis of factors affecting their
    incidence. Br J Anaes 1993; 71: 517–522
Palazzo M, Evans R. Logistic regression analysis of fixed patient factors for postoperative
    sickness: a model for risk assessment. Br J Anaes 1993; 70: 135–140
Watcha M F, White P F. Postoperative nausea and vomiting: its etiology, treatment and
    prevention. Anesthesiology 1992; 77: 162–184
Palazzo M G A, Strunin L. Anaesthesia and emesis I: etiology. Can Anaes Soc J 1984;
    31: 178–187
Palazzo M G A, Strunin L. Anaesthesia and emesis II: prevention and management. Can
    Anaes Soc J 1984: 31: 407–415
Strunin L. How long should patients fast before surgery? Time for new guidelines. Br J
    Anaes 1993; 70: 1–3

A previously healthy 38-year-old man underwent a tibial nailing for a fracture sustained during a motor cycle accident. He did not receive pre-medication, and a rapid sequence induction was performed using alfentanil, thiopentone and suxamethonium. Endotracheal intubation was accomplished and anaesthesia maintained with isoflurane in nitrous oxide and oxygen. Morphine was administered and muscle relaxation obtained with atracurium. The inspired anaesthetic gas mixture was delivered via a circle system and low flows (less than 1 L/min) were used from 15 minutes after induction.

Forty-five minutes later the end tidal CO_2 began to rise from 4.5 kPa and within 30 minutes was 8 kPa. This was accompanied by tachycardia and hypertension but oxygenation remained satisfactory. The patient was flushed and warm to touch. Immediate action included a return to high gas flows with 100% oxygen, increasing minute ventilation and discontinuing the isoflurane. It was noted that no CO_2 cylinder was attached to the anaesthetic machine. An arterial blood sample was taken for analysis and a nasopharyngeal temperature probe was placed revealing a value of 37.1°C. The arterial blood sample gave the following values: pH 7.30; PaO_2 33.2 kPa; $PaCO_2$ 9.3 kPa and HCO_3 30 mmol/l.

An electrolyte screen on the same sample demonstrated normal values. The end-tidal CO_2 analyser was therefore deemed to be functioning correctly. By this time, the end-tidal CO_2 reading was falling and isoflurane and nitrous oxide were reintroduced. A systematic check of the breathing system demonstrated a change in colour of the absorber within the circle, and the canister was warm to touch. The operation was successfully concluded and the absorber changed with no problems with subsequent cases.

DISCUSSION POINTS

Increasing carbon dioxide tensions under general anaesthesia fall into one or more of four categories: inadvertent administration of the gas; an increase in carbon dioxide production; a failure to remove expired carbon dioxide and a failure of the monitoring equipment.

- **Question 1:** *Can you discuss the differential diagnosis of an acute rise in the measured end-tidal CO_2 in an anaesthetised patient?*

Carbon dioxide cylinders are not present on all anaesthetic machines. There have been incidents where patients have been harmed by the inadvertent administration of carbon dioxide.

- **Question 2:** *Do you think that the advantages of its availability outweigh the potential hazards?*

With the widespread introduction of capnography, many anaesthetists have come to rely on this as an accurate and reliable predictor of arterial pCO_2. However, the arterial-end tidal CO_2 gradient is influenced by many factors and may be unexpectedly large or even negative. The inspired CO_2 as recorded on a capnograph may not increase despite rebreathing.

- **Question 3:** *Can you discuss the reasons for this? It is wise to confirm any unexpected findings with arterial blood gas analysis.*

FURTHER READING

Baker A B. Low-flow and closed circuits. Anaesth Intensive Care 1994; 22: 341–342 (and following articles)
Bruce W. Anaesthetic breathing systems. In: Scientific foundations of anaesthesia and intensive care. 4th edition. London: Heinmann Medical, 1990: 673–687

Weingarten M. Respiratory monitoring of carbon dioxide and oxygen; a ten-year perspective. J Clin Monitoring 1990; 6: 217–225

Riley R H et al. Detection of a faulty carbon dioxide absorber by capnography. Anaesth Intensive Care 1992; 20: 246

Nunn J F. Carbon dioxide cylinders on anaesthetic apparatus. Br J Anaes 1990; 65: 155–156

Adams A P. Capnography and pulse oximetry. In: Atkinson and Adams, eds. Recent advances in anaesthesia and analgesia. Edinburgh: Churchill Livingstone, 1989: vol 16: 155–175

Connective tissue disease

A 50-year-old man was admitted to the medical ward with a 4-month history of slowly developing angina, sweating and loss of weight. He had been previously well, was a non-smoker and drank only moderate amounts of alcohol. Small raised, red marks had recently appeared on his arms and legs.

On examination he was pale and had obviously lost weight. His blood pressure was elevated at 180/90 mmHg and heart rate was 110/min. The lesions on his arms and legs appeared vasculitic in nature. Polyarteritis nodosa was considered as a possible diagnosis and when the full blood count revealed a leucocytosis and eosinophilia, steroids were commenced as first-line treatment. Initially his symptoms appeared to settle but the following day he developed severe abdominal pain. A laparotomy was performed at which a portion of ischaemic small bowel involved in the disease process was resected. The remainder of the bowel appeared viable and simple resection with primary anastomosis was carried out.

An intravenous feeding catheter was inserted in the right subclavian vein in order to provide access for total parenteral nutrition post-operatively. The urine output was poor in the immediate postoperative period and a moderately high central venous pressure was maintained with fluid and a dopamine infusion was commenced. Despite these measures both urea and creatinine increased overnight, although urine output increased.

The following evening his condition deteriorated further when he developed severe abdominal pain, his blood pressure fell and temperature increased. Plasma protein solution was given, the infusion rate of dopa-mine increased and a further laparotomy planned. The anaesthetist on this occasion felt his condition warranted invasive blood pressure monitoring but because his peripheral arterial blood supply was already critical, an arterial line was not inserted. After pre-oxygenation, anaesthesia was induced with thiopentone and alfentanil, cricoid pressure applied and suxamethonium was used to facilitate endotracheal intubation. Anaesthesia was maintained with isoflurane in oxygen and nitrous oxide and fentanyl was given for analgesia. Muscle relaxation was maintained with atracurium. At laparotomy it was necessary to resect almost the entire small bowel because of thrombosis and resulting ischaemia. Post-operatively he was transferred to ITU.

The pathology report from the first laparotomy stated that there were multiple small nodules characteristic of polyarteritis nodosa on the smaller arteries. The vessel walls were infiltrated by polymorphs and there was evidence of necrosis with resultant aneurysmal dilatation.

DISCUSSION POINTS

This patient was male, with recent onset of disease, and life-threatening consequences of polyarteritis nodosa.

- *Question 1:* *Can you describe the main features of this connective tissue disease?*

- *Question 2:* *What other connective tissue disease patterns are commonly encountered and what are the characteristics features of these?*

Total parenteral nutrition is used commonly in seriously ill patients.

- *Question 3:* *How would you determine the composition of the feed?*

- *Question 4:* *Enteral feeding is preferred in most circumstances. Why is this so? What are the benefits to the patient of enteral as opposed to parenteral feeding?*

Invasive arterial pressure monitoring is widely used with relatively few complications.

● *Question 5: In what situations would you avoid inserting an arterial line?*

● *Question 6: What complications can arise and what is their incidence?*

This patient had recently commenced steroid treatment. Other patients may present having been on long-term steroid treatment, or having recently discontinued a course of steroid treatment.

● *Question 7: How would you manage steroid therapy in these groups of patients, and what are the potential problems?*

FURTHER READING

When the lungs are involved by connective tissue disease. Postgraduate Medicine 1993; 94: 147–152, 154, 157–8

Davies S R. Systemic lupus erythematosus and the obstetrical patient – implications for the anaesthetist. Can J Anaes 1991; 38: 790–796

Haynes B F, Allen N B, Fauci A S. Diagnostic and therapeutic approach to the patient with vasculitis. Medical Clinics of North America. Advances in Rheumatology 1986; 70: 355–368

du Bois R M. Pathogenetic mechanism in the lung in systemic disease. Postgraduate Medical J 1988; 64(supp 4): 103–110

Salem M, Tanish Jr R E, Bromberg J, Loriaux D L, Chernow B. Perioperative glucocorticoid coverage: a reassessment 42 years after emergence of a problem. Ann Surg 1994; 219: 416–425

Sax H C, Souba W W. Enteral and parenteral feedings: guidelines and recommendations. Medical Clinics of North America 1993; 77: 863–880

15 Hepatic dysfunction

A 60-year-old woman was admitted to the gynaecological ward for further investigation and management of bilateral ovarian masses and ascites seen on ultrasound at an outpatient clinic. There was a 6-month history of general malaise and more recently of increasing weight and abdominal swelling. Initial routine blood investigations are shown in Table 1; an ECG demonstrated inferolateral ischaemic changes, and a chest X-ray displayed a right upper lobe consolidation (Fig. 15.1). General examination was consistent with ascites and a chest infection and bilateral pitting oedema of her legs to upper thigh was apparent. She was commenced on spironolactone, vitamin K and intravenous antibiotics.

Two days after admission she complained of increasing breathlessness, and examination revealed tachypnoea (26/min) and tachycardia (106/min), a blood pressure of 100/70 mmHg and a temperature of 38°C. A further chest X-ray demonstrated the development of gas under the diaphragm. Emergency surgery was planned involving both gynaecology staff and general surgeons because of the likelihood of bowel perforation. She was reviewed pre-operatively by the anaesthetist, who ascertained she had never been in hospital before and was on no medication before this hospital admission. In light of the blood results indicating significant

Table 1 Blood results

Results	On admission	Postop	48 h postop
Na	139	137	158
K	3.3	4.3	3.9
BIC	28	17	23
urea	3.9	10.1	29.3
creat	89	144	231
albumin	18	29	26
bilirubin	24	172	260
AAT	48	76	150
GGT	181	86	100
PT	25.3	–	–
APTT	63.4	–	–
TCT	29	–	–

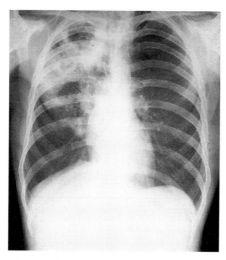

Fig. 15.1 Chest X-ray showing RUL consolidation with cavitation

liver impairment and a coagulopathy, 4 units of fresh-frozen plasma were made available and 6 units of blood were cross-matched.

On arrival in the anaesthetic room basic monitoring was established, two 14-G cannulae were inserted with local anaesthesia and the patient was pre-oxygenated. Infusion of the fresh-frozen plasma was completed during this time. A rapid sequence induction of anaesthesia was performed with etomidate, suxamethonium and alfentanil. After checking correct insertion of the endotracheal tube, anaesthesia was maintained with isoflurane and nitrous oxide in oxygen supplemented with fentanyl. Atracurium provided further muscle relaxation. Before transfer to theatre direct arterial pressure monitoring was established and a central line was inserted. During the procedure, all fluids were warmed and the upper body was covered with a heated air warmer.

The laparotomy confirmed bilateral ovarian masses and ascites and revealed the source of the peritoneal air was a perforation in the sigmoid colon with extensive left sided abscess formation. Other findings were a large cirrhotic liver with extensive varicoele formation and splenomegaly. During the laparotomy the sigmoid and left colon were mobilised with considerable difficulty and considerable blood loss due to the long-standing abscess.

Macroscopic examination of the removed colon revealed extensive diverticular disease. A colostomy was fashioned at the right upper quadrant. Both ovaries were removed and sent with the excised colon for pathological examination.

Blood loss during the procedure was estimated as 5000 ml and in total 7500 ml of fluid was given, including 9 units of concentrated red cells and

6 units of cryoprecipitate in addition to the 4 units of fresh-frozen plasma. Once surgery was completed the abdomen was packed with proflavine-soaked packs and the patient transferred to the intensive care unit. Although there was no evidence of bleeding at the end of the procedure, it was thought prudent in light of the coagulopathy and extensive bleeding during this procedure to re-examine the abdominal cavity after a period of stabilisation and further correction of blood indices.

On arrival in the intensive care unit further blood sampling was performed and a pulmonary artery catheter was inserted. Inotropic support with low-dose dopamine and adrenaline was required over the following 48 hours to maintain blood pressure and optimise oxygen delivery. Re-examination of the abdomen 36 hours later revealed no further evidence of bleeding when the packs were removed and the abdomen was closed. Despite optimisation with inotropes, guided by the pulmonary artery catheter measurements, she developed increasing renal impairment (Table 1). Diuretic therapy was commenced with spironolactone and then supplemented with frusemide and urine output improved. Over the following week renal function continued to improve and inotropic support was gradually withdrawn. One week after admission to the intensive care unit the cirrhosis was diagnosed as secondary to primary biliary cirrhosis, when results of auto-antibody tests revealed a high smooth muscle antibody titre.

DISCUSSION POINTS

The patient with moderate or severe liver disease is at high risk from surgery, anaesthesia, or trauma. However, due to the large reserve of the liver, there will usually not be clinical evidence of hepatic pathology until at least 70% of the functional liver mass is lost. Child's classification with later addition of the prothrombin time by Pugh has been the standard for assessing surgical risk and hepatic reserve. Patients are divided into low, moderate and high risk groups. This patient was in a high risk group and as a result of that her risk of mortality from surgery was more than 50%.

- *Question 1: Describe the signs of hepatic failure which may be found on physical examination.*

- **Question 2:** *Describe the blood and oxygen supply to the liver. How will this change during low flow or hypoxaemic events?*

- **Question 3:** *Outline the cardiovascular and pulmonary abnormalities in the patient with cirrhosis and liver failure.*

- **Question 4:** *Is monitoring with a pulmonary artery catheter of value in the patient with liver failure undergoing resuscitation? How would the typically measured indices vary from the normal patient?*

Electrolyte abnormalities are common in patients with liver failure, with the accumulation of intravascular and interstitial fluid. Alkalotic hypokalaemia and high total body sodium are seen commonly.

- **Question 5:** *Outline the mechanisms which result in this, and describe what therapy might be appropriate.*

The patient with alcoholic liver disease may have resistance to sedative drugs, e.g. opioids, at an early stage of his or her disease, yet at a later stage be extremely sensitive.

• **Question 6:** *Discuss management of postoperative pain control in the patient at these two stages, considering the risks and benefits of opioid analgesia and regional techniques.*

Renal failure is a serious complication found in patients with hepatic failure subjected to stressful events such as haemorrhage or surgery.

• **Question 7:** *Discuss the mechanisms possible in this development.*

• **Question 8:** *How would you attempt to minimise the risk?*

FURTHER READING

Gelman S. Anaesthesia and the liver. In: Barash P G, Cullen B F, Steotling R K, Clinical anaesthesia. 2nd ed. Philadelphia: JB Lippencott, 1992: 1185–1214
Gomez G A, Jacobson L E, Asensio J A, Nuata R J. Pre-existing liver disease in the trauma patient. Trauma and pre-existing disease, Part II: Specific management concerns. Critical Care Medicine 1994; 10: 555–566

16 Asthma

A 32-year-old woman was admitted to the acute surgical ward with a 12-hour history of anorexia and abdominal pain which had originally been central in origin but was now mostly felt in her right iliac fossa. Her temperature was 38°C and on examination of the abdomen there was marked right iliac fossa tenderness with guarding. Her full blood count showed a white count of 13×10^4 and urinalysis was negative. A diagnosis of acute appendicitis was made and surgery proposed.

Her past medical history consisted of asthma since childhood. Current medication consisted of salbutamol and beclomethasone inhalers four times daily. Two years previously a chest infection precipitated an acute exacerbation of her asthma necessitating hospital admission and treatment with nebulised salbutamol and intravenous hydrocortisone and aminophylline. She had required no steroid therapy since and considered her condition presently under good control. Peak expiratory flow rate two days earlier had been 410/min.

The anaesthetist found her to be slightly obese with a respiratory rate of 20 breaths/min. Although not complaining of dyspnoea, auscultation revealed mild generalised rhonchi and she was asked to use her inhalers prior to transfer to theatre.

In the anaesthetic room intravenous access was secured and basic monitoring established. A rapid sequence intravenous induction with thiopentone and suxamethonium was performed following pre-oxygenation. The trachea was intubated and her lungs were ventilated with isoflurane in 100% oxygen until correct tracheal tube position was confirmed and it was ascertained there was no leak round the cuff. Anaesthesia was maintained with isoflurane and nitrous oxide in oxygen supplemented with fentanyl and droperidol. Vecuronium provided further muscle relaxation.

While the patient was being further prepared for transfer into the operating theatre, it was noticed that the airway inflation pressure had increased to 60 cm H_2O. Oxygen saturation readings on the pulse oximeter fell from 99% to 90%. Auscultation revealed equal air entry with widespread inspiratory and expiratory wheeze throughout the chest. A suction catheter passed through the endotracheal tube revealed no evidence of obstruction and obtained only a small volume of clear sputum. The systolic blood pressure remained at 120 mmHg. Nitrous oxide was discontinued, anaesthesia deepened with isoflurane and aminophylline and hydrocortisone were administered intravenously. Despite these measures there was little improvement, salbutamol was administered by slow intra-venous injection and this was followed by a slow fall in inflation pressure and rise in oxygen saturation. A chest X-ray was performed to rule out pneumothorax. When the chest X-ray had been checked the situation appeared to have resolved and the patient was transferred to theatre where an inflamed appendix was removed without further incident.

In the recovery room she again became wheezy. This was treated with nebulised salbutamol. Further questioning of the patient later revealed a history of a mild upper respiratory tract infection two weeks previously.

DISCUSSION POINTS

There will be limited time available for the pre-operative assessment and preparation of an asthmatic patient presenting as a surgical emergency. Many of the useful investigations are effort-dependant (e.g. peak flow measurements, spirometry) and the results may be meaningless in the patient with an acute abdomen. Recent investigations, history and the patients' assessment of their current respiratory status may be more helpful.

- *Question 1:* *Outline the features of note in this patient's presentation and discuss the relevance of the recent upper respiratory tract infection.*

- *Question 2:* *Describe the pathophysiology and rationale of therapy in an acute exacerbation of asthma.*

Pre-oxygenation is carried out prior to a rapid sequence intravenous induction and in other patients thought to be at risk of hypoxia at the time of intubation.

- **Question 3:** *What are the aims of pre-oxygenation and for how long should it be carried out?*

- **Question 4:** *Will this vary in patients with obstructive airways disease?*

Chronic respiratory disease is commonly encountered in patients presenting for surgery. Pulmonary function tests can help identify whether lung disease is of an obstructive or restrictive pattern, quantify the extent of the disease, determine the response to therapy and monitor the rate of progress.

- **Question 5:** *What measurements are made in pulmonary function testing and how will these vary from the norm in both obstructive and restrictive disease?*

FURTHER READING

Hirshman C A. Peri-operative management of the asthmatic patient. Can J Anaes 1991; 38: 4 R26–R32
Barnes P J. A new approach to the treatment of asthma. N Eng J Med 1989; 321: 1517–27
British Thoracic Society. Guidelines for the management of asthma in adults: II – acute severe asthma. BMJ 1990; 301: 797–800
Campbell I T, Beatty P C W. Monitoring pre-oxygenation. Br J Anaes 1994; 72: 3–4
Zibrak J D, O'Donnell C R, Marton K I. Pre-operative pulmonary function testing (position paper). American College of Physicians. Ann Int Med 1990; 112: 793–794

17 Renal transplant

A 32-year-old woman with a 3-year history of renal failure requiring haemodialysis was admitted for renal transplantation. Renal failure was secondary to a 20-year history of insulin-dependant diabetes. When seen pre-operatively she had just been dialysed for 3 hours. She said she was a little anxious about the anaesthesia, but more so about the possible disappointment ahead should the transplant prove unsuccessful. Her obesity was noted by the anaesthetist (weight 84 kg, height 150 cm) and possibilities for venous access seemed poor. There was an arteriovenous shunt on her right arm. A previous shunt on the left arm had failed 6 months previously. Full blood count, urea and electrolytes and blood glucose results were available (Table 1). Two units of blood were cross-matched.

Before coming to theatre an intravenous infusion of 4% glucose and 0.9% saline was commenced at 80 ml/hr with an actrapid insulin infusion according to BM stix estimation of blood glucose. This continued throughout the procedure and thereafter into the post-operative period until normal nutrition was established. Premedication consisted of ranitidine orally and heparin subcutaneously. Her right arm was wrapped loosely in cotton wool to protect her arteriovenous fistula.

In the anaesthetic room after establishing basic monitoring, azathioprine, hydrocortisone and cefuroxime were given intravenously. Following pre-oxygenation, anaesthesia was induced with thiopentone and morphine. Atracurium provided muscle relaxation permitting successful intubation, and anaesthesia was maintained with isoflurane and nitrous oxide in oxygen.

Table 1 Blood results

Electrolytes	Immediately pre-operatively	12 h postop
Na	133	139
K	5.7	7.0
bicarbonate	18	17
urea	12.9	14.5
creatinine	596	652
glucose	10.1	9.8
haemoglobin	8.4	7.9

Surgery proved awkward due to the patient's size and the procedure took over three hours to complete instead of the expected two. She was cardiovascularly stable throughout. Prior to completion of the anastomosis to the transplanted kidney she received 1.75 L of crystalloid. As the anastomosis was completed methylprednisolone and mannitol were given intravenously.

Only 23 ml of urine was passed during the remainder of the procedure; however, the kidney looked viable and surgery was completed. Postoperative fluids were initially prescribed at a rate of 100 ml/h, and analgesia was provided by means of a morphine patient controlled analgesia pump.

Overnight, little urine was passed despite fluid challenges and increasing the background rate of intravenous fluid administration. Ultrasound investigation of the kidney the following morning suggested no urinary obstruction, but little evidence of blood flow within the transplanted organ. On examination she was thought to be mildly oedematous and following electrolyte measurement it was apparent she required further haemodialysis Table 1. The acutely-rejected kidney was later removed at a second laparotomy. She remains on twice weekly haemodialysis, awaiting a second organ donation.

DISCUSSION POINTS

In 1959 brain death was described by Mollaret and Goulon in France and formally accepted in the United Kingdom in 1976. Although the aim of this description was to prevent unnecessary therapy in the face of a hopeless prognosis, the diagnosis has since permitted the use of organs from beating-heart donors. Good donor maintenance before and during organ donation is essential for optimal function of transplanted organs.

● *Question 1:* *Detail the criteria for establishing the diagnosis of brainstem death in the United Kingdom.*

● **Question 2:** *Outline the management of the multiple organ donor, up to and including the removal of organs.*

Surgical access was thought to be impeded by this patient's obesity. In addition, venous access was noted by the anaesthetist to be poor. This could have been due to her diabetic condition, her renal failure, but also influenced by her obesity.

● **Question 3:** *Describe the pathophysiology of the morbidly obese patient, and the peri-operative anaesthetic management of such a patient.*

The prime regulatory organ for potassium homeostasis is the kidney, until acute renal failure or advanced chronic renal failure supervenes. Homeostasis of potassium, as the principal intracellular ion, is vital for normal function of the body.

● **Question 4:** *Describe the changes in potassium regulation as renal failure develops.*

● **Question 5:** *What are the presenting features of hyperkalaemia and hypokalaemia, and what is the mechanism behind their development?*

- **Question 6:** *Discuss the pre-operative assessment and preparation of the patient with chronic renal failure.*

- **Question 7:** *Discuss the influence of the anaesthetic technique on the success of renal transplantation.*

- **Question 8:** *Do you consider the monitoring in this case was optimal?*

FURTHER READING

The organ donor. The Intensive Care Society, London 1994

Bodenham A, Park G R. Care of the multiple organ donor. Intensive Care Med 1989; 15: 340–348

Pallis C. Diagnosis of brain stem death. ABC of brain stem death. BMJ 1982; 285: 1558–1560, 1641–1644, 1720–1722

Tetzlaff J E, O'Hara Jr. J F, Walsh M T. Potassium and anaesthesia. Can J Anaes 1993; 40: 227–246

Chronic renal failure. Practitioner. January 1993; 237: 1522, 1564–69

Shenkman Z, Shir Y, Brodsky J B. Peri-operative management of the obese patient. Br J Anaes 1993; 70: 349–359

18 Collapse during laparoscopy

A 37-year-old female underwent laparoscopy and hydrotubation on a day-case basis as part of the investigation of secondary infertility. She was otherwise healthy and prepared for general anaesthesia. In the anaesthetic room basic monitoring was established and a 20 G cannula inserted in the dorsum of the hand. Anaesthesia was induced with fentanyl, droperidol and propofol. Vecuronium was administered to facilitate tracheal intubation and intermittent positive pressure ventilation was commenced with isoflurane in 66% nitrous oxide and oxygen.

The patient was then transferred to theatre and placed in the lithotomy position with a head-down tilt. The surgeon introduced the Verres' needle and carbon dioxide was insufflated to produce a pneumoperitoneum. After the insufflation of about 3 L, the ECG and pulse oximeter alarm showed a sinus bradycardia of 35/min. The non-invasive blood pressure monitor was unable to produce a reading. The surgeon discontinued the insufflation and released gas from the abdomen, although the intra-abdominal pressure reading did not appear excessively high. Meanwhile the anaesthetist discontinued the volatile agent, continued IPPV with 100% oxygen and gave atropine intravenously. The anaesthetic assistant removed the head-down tilt. The pulse rate decreased no further and increased to 60/min within 90 seconds. The blood pressure monitor gave a reading of 80/50 mmHg at the next cycle, and one minute later read 90/60 mmHg.

After the anaesthetist was satisfied that the patient's condition was stable and satisfactory for 5 minutes, surgery again proceeded, this time without adverse event. As the procedure finished anaesthesia was discontinued, and once spontaneous respiration was adequate the patient was extubated and transferred to the recovery room. Her postoperative recordings remained satisfactory.

DISCUSSION POINTS

The initial response to this critical incident under general anaesthesia was to attempt to restore circulation as soon as possible no matter the exact mechanism of the collapse. The volatile agent was discontinued and IPPV continued with 100% oxygen, the surgical stimulus removed and an anticholinergic agent administered. Had this not resolved the situation immediately, or had the pulse rate continued to decrease, then external cardiac massage would have commenced and the patient returned to the supine position.

● **Question 1:** *Discuss the possible mechanisms for the critical incident in this case with reference to the anaesthetic technique employed and the surgery being undertaken.*

● **Question 2:** *What other forms of monitoring might have been useful in this situation?*

● **Question 3:** *Why is carbon dioxide used to create the pneumoperitoneum at laparoscopy? Discuss how this may influence the anaesthetic technique.*

Laparoscopic techniques are being used increasingly by general surgeons for a variety of techniques, but experience is greatest for laparoscopic cholecystectomy.

● **Question 4:** *Outline the benefits for the patient of laparoscopic cholecystectomy as opposed to open cholecystectomy.*

- **Question 5:** *Outline the cardiovascular and respiratory effects on the patient of the Trendelenberg position.*

FURTHER READING

Cunningham A J, Brull S J. Laparoscopic cholecystectomy: anaesthetic implications. Anaes Analg 1993; 76: 1120–1133

Hanley E S. Anaesthesia for laparoscopic surgery. Surgical Clinics of North America 1992; 72: 1013–1019

Shilman H D, Aronson H B. Capnography in the early diagnosis of CO_2 embolism during laparoscopy. Can Anaes Soc J 1984; 31: 455–459

Whitwam J G. Minimally invasive therapy implications for anaesthesia. Anaesthesia 1993; 48: 937–939

Coventry D M, McMenemin I, Lawrie S. Bradycardias during intra-abdominal surgery: Modification by pre-operative anti-cholinergic agents. Anaesthesia 1987; 42: 835–9

Cardiac tamponade

A 70-year-old man underwent aortic valve replacement with a mechanical valve for post-rheumatic aortic stenosis. He was discharged after 7 days but re-admitted 4 days later complaining of increasing shortness of breath and general malaise and central chest pain on coughing or deep inspiration. His current medication was frusemide and warfarin but his INR had not been measured since discharge. On examination he was mildly dyspnoeic at rest with bilateral basal crepitations and raised jugulo-venous pressure with marked systolic descent. He had bilateral pitting ankle oedema and his liver was enlarged two finger-breadths and tender. Chest X-ray showed generally plethoric lung fields and although his heart was enlarged, this was not a new finding. In addition the sternal edges were mobile on palpation and the lower end of his wound was erythematous. A diagnosis of congestive cardiac failure with sternal dehiscence was made. Intravenous frusemide brought a subjective improvement in his symptoms, although his JVP remained elevated. He required re-suture of his sternum, and when seen by the anaesthetist, his symptomatology had much improved and his chest was clear. The INR was 6 and the surgeon was happy to proceed provided 2 units of fresh-frozen plasma were given.

The following morning, he received temazepam as pre-medication. During pre-oxygenation a radial artery line was placed under local anaesthesia revealing a systolic blood pressure of 110 mmHg and heart rate of 90/min. During induction of anaesthesia he received alfentanil, thiopentone and vecuronium. The blood pressure fell to 70 mmHg and heart rate increased to 120/min. Despite rapid intubation and ventilation with an F_1O_2 of 1.0, the blood pressure continued to fall. His legs were elevated, he was given methoxamine, phenylephrine and then adrenaline but the blood pressure remained at 50 mmHg systolic and heart rate was 130/min. By this time the situation was grave with an unresponsive low blood pressure and oxygen saturation of 70%. As external cardiac massage was instituted, the surgeon was called urgently to open the previous incision and this produced a sudden gush of a few hundred ml of blood. This almost immediately restored the blood pressure and oxygen saturation. Thereafter the operation proceeded uneventfully but recovery was prolonged with a period of postoperative confusion which lasted 24 hours.

DISCUSSION POINTS

This was a case of missed diagnosis.

- *Question 1: What clinical features were present pre-operatively which suggested the possibility of cardiac tamponade?*

- *Question 2: What further investigation might have confirmed the diagnosis pre-operatively?*

- *Question 3: What features of the arterial trace, if looked for, might have suggested the presence of tamponade?*

- *Question 4: Had the diagnosis been established earlier, what further procedure might have avoided cardiovascular collapse during induction of anaesthesia?*

● **Question 5:** *Cardiac tamponade may occur early or late after cardiac surgery. List other common causes of cardiac tamponade.*

● **Question 6:** *Describe the physiology of tamponade and the effects of positive pressure ventilation in this situation.*

FURTHER READING

Muir J, Wilkowski D A. The pericardium and anaesthesia. In: Tarhan S, ed. Cardiovascular anaesthesia and postoperative care. Yearbook Medical Publishers Inc 2nd edn 1989: 301–327

Fowler N. Cardiac tamponade – a clinical or an echocardiographic diagnosis? Circulation 1993; 87: 1738–1741

Shwartz S L, Pandian N G, Cao Q, Hsu T, et al. Left ventricular diastolic collapse in regional left heart cardiac tamponade. An experimental echocardiographic and haemodynamic study. JACC 1993; 22: 907–913

Devitt J N, McLean R F, McLellan, B A. Perioperative cardiovascular complications associated with blunt thoracic trauma. Can J Anaes 1993; 40: 197–200

20 Subarachnoid haemorrhage

A 23-year-old 68 kg male in a conscious but drowsy and disorientated condition was taken to the Accident and Emergency Department following a collapse at home. He complained of a severe headache which was exacerbated by the bright lights of the admission room. On examination his clothing was soiled with vomit, he had been incontinent and his peripheral temperature was recorded as 38.2°C. He was noted to have neural rigidity and to be hypertensive with a blood pressure of 200/120 mmHg. An ECG showed ST elevation in lead I and aVL, with evidence of left ventricular hypertrophy and strain in the chest leads. As a child the patient had been extensively investigated for failure to thrive, but no diagnosis had ever been reached. With this exception there was no past medical history of note. A diagnosis of probable subarachnoid haemorrhage (SAH) was made and the patient was commenced on an infusion of nimodipine. The diagnosis was later confirmed with a CT scan which showed haemorrhage from the left-middle cerebral artery.

Following admission the patient's hypertension gave considerable cause for concern and he was started on an infusion of labetalol. His blood pressure was subsequently controlled at 150/85 mmHg. Review of the chest X-ray revealed not only cardiomegaly, but also rib notching, raising the suspicion of a coincidental aortic coarctation (Fig. 20.1). Femoral catheterisation was not possible and cerebral angiography was achieved by

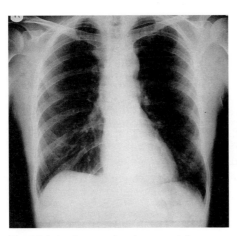

Fig. 20.1 Angiogram showing coarctation

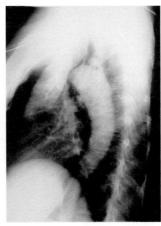

Fig. 20.2 Chest X-ray showing rib notching

cannulation of the left axillary artery. This confirmed the presence of an aneurysm of the left middle cerebral artery. An aortic coarctation measuring 3.5 cm in length was also demonstrated at the time of cerebral angiography just distal to the left subclavian artery together with a well-developed collateral system (Fig. 20.2).

In view of the coexisting aortic coarctation and as this was a middle cerebral aneurysm, with a significant chance of early re-bleeding, definitive aneurysmal clipping was proposed and the patient underwent surgery 2 days after admission.

Temazepam was given orally as premedication one hour prior to surgery. In the anaesthetic room basic monitoring and invasive blood pressure recording were established. Anaesthesia was induced with fentanyl and thiopentone and suxamethonium was given to facilitate tracheal intubation. Anaesthesia was maintained with isoflurane in 50% nitrous oxide in oxygen and atracurium was given to provide further neuromuscular blockade. Surgery proceeded uneventfully for the first 2 hours, but despite the systolic blood pressure being maintained at approximately 20 mmHg below the induction level of 155/85 mmHg, the aneurysm ruptured intra-operatively. Rapid hypotension was induced and with this, and the use of temporary clips on adjacent vessels, clipping of the aneurysm was achieved. The postoperative course was complicated by vasospasm, but eventual recovery was satisfactory with only mild residual sensory aphasia and a degree of emotional lability.

Three months later, the patient was admitted for surgery to correct the aortic coarctation. This was undertaken with the use of a Gott shunt without the need for cardiopulmonary bypass, and following a short period of convalescence the patient made an uncomplicated recovery.

DISCUSSION POINTS

Timing of cerebral aneurysm surgery is controversial. One large international study has shown the incidence of rebleeding in good grade patients (alert) to be lower if surgery is performed within 3 days of SAH rather then later surgery (day 7–day 11). The mortality was not influenced by the timing of surgery. However, in the North American subset of this study best results were obtained in the group with early surgery. Following SAH the two critical events that prejudice a favourable outcome are rebleeding and vasospasm. Nimodipine has recently been introduced to attempt to reduce the incidence of vasospasm.

- **Question 1:** *Describe what kind of an agent nimodipine is, how it can be administered, and what the proposed mechanism of action is.*

- **Question 2:** *What are the risks of nimodipine interacting with anaesthetic agents?*

- **Question 3:** *In order to reduce risks of bleeding there are occasions when the blood pressure is lowered. Would this be considered in this patient and would there be any problems in doing so?*

- **Question 4:** *What type of monitoring would be required for this patient during this surgery, bearing in mind the existing coarctation?*

Induction of anaesthesia represents a critical period for the patient with an unsecured cerebral aneurysm. The goal is to achieve a smooth induction while maintaining normal or slightly reduced aneurysmal transmural pressure.

- *Question 5:* *Do you consider that the timing of monitoring and the agents used in this case appropriate?*

- *Question 6:* *Would other techniques and drugs have been as appropriate, or superior?*

- *Question 7:* *Mannitol is used during neurosurgery to reduce cerebral swelling. How does this affect fluid management in patients during and after the surgery?*

Rapid hypotension was required following intra-operative aneurysm rupture to facilitate optimum surgical conditions.

- *Question 8:* *What agents are commonly used for this purpose?*

- *Question 9:* *What are the pharmacological actions of these agents?*

FURTHER READING

Kazuo Abe. Vasodilators during cerebral aneurysm surgery. Can J Anaes 1993; 40: 775–90

Archer D A, Leblanc R L. Haemodynamic considerations in the management of patients with subarachnoid haemorrhage. Can J Anaes 1991; 38: 454–70

Nimodipine for delayed cerebral ischaemia after subarachnoid haemorrhage. Drugs and Therapeutics Bulletin. Oct 1992; 39: 81–3

Merin R G. Calcium channel-blocking drugs and anaesthetics. Is the drug interaction beneficial or detrimental? Anesthesiology 1987; 66: 111–3

Hollier L H. Protecting the brain and spinal cord. J Vascular Surg 1987; 5: 534–8

Herrick I A, Gelb A W. Anesthesia for intracranial aneurysm surgery. J Clinical Anes Jan–Feb 1992; 4: 73–85

Lam A M, Mayberg T S. Use of nitrous oxide in neuroanesthesia: why bother? J Neurosurg Anes 1992; 4: 285–89

Samra S K. Place of nitrous oxide in neuroanesthesia: still a valuable drug. J Neurosurg Anes 1992; 4: 290–94

21 Brain biopsy

A 12-year-old boy was diagnosed as having neurofibromatosis after referral to a dermatology clinic. One year later he attended the neurology clinic complaining of headaches. A CT scan of the brain performed at this time revealed two small lesions in the paravertebral area. Two months later he was admitted as an emergency to the neurology ward following the onset of right-sided weakness and facial paraesthesia. A second CT scan was performed that day revealing a third lesion, significant increase in the size of the two previously noted lesions, and some compression of the ventricular system. Stereotactic biopsy of these lesions was scheduled two days hence.

A pre-operative visit revealed that the child had been well until recently. Other medical history included removal of adenoids and tonsils six years previously, with no anaesthetic problems. Examination did not reveal any new physical findings.

It was planned to anaesthetise the child in theatre and apply the stereotactic frame. He would then be transferred to the CT scan room to establish the co-ordinates required for biopsy and then return to theatre for surgery.

After an overnight fast, EMLA cream was applied to both hands 90 minutes before coming to theatre. After basic monitoring was established, a 20-gauge intravenous cannula was inserted to the dorsum of one hand. Induction of anaesthesia proceeded with propofol and lignocaine. He was manually hyperventilated with oxygen, then lignocaine, alfentanil and atracurium were given. Neuromuscular blockade was confirmed and the trachea easily intubated. After checking correct endotracheal tube position, the tube was carefully fastened and the patient was ventilated with oxygen-enriched air. Anaesthesia was maintained with a computer-controlled infusion of propofol and incremental doses of alfentanil. Neuromuscular blockade was maintained with atracurium and a larger-bore venous cannula and radial arterial line were inserted.

The surgeon infiltrated the skin with local anaesthetic and then applied the frame. The child was then connected to portable monitoring equipment and ventilator. The child was transferred to the CT scan room where it took 20 minutes to perform the scan. He was then transferred back to theatre, and when the co-ordinates became available three biopsies were performed through two burr holes.

As the bandage was applied the propofol infusion was discontinued and muscle paralysis reversed with neostigmine and glycopyrrolate. After the return of spontaneous respiration, he was transferred onto his bed and extubated on his side. He was transferred back to the ward after a short uneventful period in the recovery room.

DISCUSSION POINTS

Raised intracranial pressure may develop secondary to head trauma, space occupying lesions, cerebral spinal fluid regulation problems or a mixed group, e.g. hepatic encephalopathy or malignant hypertension. This may ultimately result in herniation of the cerebellum through the foramen magnum and compression of the medulla ('coning').

● *Question 1: Describe the compensatory mechanisms that may have taken place before this catastrophic event when raised intracranial pressure develops slowly.*

In the presence of space-occupying lesions and raised intracranial pressure, induction of anaesthesia, laryngoscopy and tracheal intubation are best performed with optimum haemodynamic stability.

● *Question 2: Can you comment on which agents should be avoided in this situation?*

● *Question 3: Is there any evidence to suggest that one opioid may be preferable to another?*

A total intravenous anaesthetic technique was used during this case.

● **Question 4:** *Describe the characteristics of propofol and atracurium which made them suitable agents to use.*

● **Question 5:** *What problems may arise with the use of such a technique?*

FURTHER READING

Marsh B, White M, Morton N, Kenny G N C. Pharmacokinetic model driven infusion of propofol in children. Br J Anaes 1991; 67: 41–48

White M, Kenny G N C. Intravenous propofol using a computerised infusion system. Anaesthesia 1990; 45: 204–209

Cohen A T. Use of alfentanil in association with intracranial disease. Anaesthesia 1993; 48: 922–923

Andrews P, Souter M. Why the eagerness to condemn? Anaesthesia 1993; 48: 1020–1

Guidelines for the transfer of critically ill patients. Guidelines of the committee of the American College of Critical Care Medicine: Society of Critical Care Medicine and the American Association of Critical Care Nurses Transfer Guidelines Task Force. J Critical Care Med 1993; 21: 931–7

Ingram G S. Neurophysiology (intracranial pressure). In: Walters, Ingram, Jenkinson, eds. Anaesthesia and intensive care for the neurosurgical patient. Oxford: Blackwell Scientific Publications, 1994

22 Post-dural puncture headache

A 60-year-old farmer was admitted for elective total hip replacement. When seen by the anaesthetist pre-operatively, the only past medical history of note was mild wheeze during the 'hay fever' season, for which he occasionally used a salbutamol inhaler. As a young man, he had had two previous general anaesthetics without problems. On examination he was found to have no abnormal physical findings. Blood pressure was measured as 130/80 mmHg. The routine pre-operative investigations of full blood count, urea and electrolytes, blood sugar, ECG and chest X-ray were found to be within normal limits. The proposed anaesthetic was discussed with the patient and it was decided to use a subarachnoid regional technique.

Premedication consisted of temazepam orally 90 minutes before the scheduled start of surgery. In the anaesthetic room, using an aseptic technique, isobaric bupivacaine 0.5% was injected into the subarachnoid space at the L3/4 interspace with a 25 G Quincke spinal needle. The procedure was uneventful and sensory anaesthesia was achieved to a level of T8 bilaterally. Intravenous midazolam was used to provide basal sedation, and he breathed oxygen-enriched air throughout the procedure. Surgery was uncomplicated. Estimated blood loss was 600 ml. Intra-operative fluids consisted of crystalloid 1500 ml and 500 ml of a synthetic colloid. He was cardiovascularly stable throughout.

Post-operative pain was controlled with the morphine delivered via a patient-controlled analgesia system. Intravenous fluids continued for the first 36 hours postoperatively and were discontinued as he started to eat and drink. Blood loss in the drains was 250 ml in the first 24 hours, and postoperative haemoglobin was 11 g/dl. He was in bed for 48 hours. On the second postoperative morning he complained of a throbbing occipital headache when he sat up to take breakfast. This settled when he took paracetamol and laid down. A few hours later, when he got up for physiotherapy for the first time, he experienced a recurrence of the headache with photophobia, nausea, dizziness and some neck stiffness. On returning to bed and lying flat the symptoms resolved.

These events were repeated the next day each time he tried to rise. In addition, he noticed occasional double vision. The surgeons were keen to mobilise the patient and so asked the anaesthetist for an opinion. A post-dural puncture headache was diagnosed. The patient was by now increasingly concerned and required reassurance from the anaesthetist. Initial advice was to continue flat bed rest for a further 24 hours with a high oral fluid intake. However, due to the patient's nausea, intravenous infusion was recommenced and 2000 ml of crystalloid was administered in this 24 hour period. In addition, the anaesthetist prescribed caffeine benzoate.

Despite this the patient still had marked symptoms when he sat up the next day. An autologous epidural blood patch was offered in view of the failure of conservative management.

Under aseptic conditions epidural puncture was performed at the L3/4 interspace using an 18 G Tuohy needle. Once the epidural space was identified, an assistant obtained 20 ml of blood from an aseptic venepuncture and the blood was injected slowly into the epidural space. During the injection the patient complained of transient neck and backache; however, very shortly after the injection his symptoms had markedly diminished. He rested in bed overnight and was able to mobilise without headache the following morning. The remainder of his hospital stay was uncomplicated.

DISCUSSION POINTS

- *Question 1: It has been said that spinal anaesthesia is 'safer' than general anaesthesia for certain patients. What evidence is there for this?*

- *Question 2: Many lower limb orthopaedic procedures are frequently performed under spinal or epidural anaesthesia. What advantages and disadvantages are there for the patients with these techniques?*

Certain patient groups are at increased risk of developing a post-dural puncture headache (PDPH). In addition, factors associated with the technique of spinal anaesthesia may influence the incidence of headache.

- **Question 3:** *Which patients have this increased risk, and how can the risks be minimised?*

- **Question 4:** *Discuss the differential diagnosis of PDPH.*

- **Question 5:** *What is the natural history of PDPH and what long-term sequelae may be experienced?*

Autologous blood patching is an effective method of treating PDPH. Studies show 89% of headaches may be cured by an initial injection of blood, and a further 8% with a second blood patch. However this is not considered the first line of management by every anaesthetist and will not be suitable for every patient.

- **Question 6:** *Outline the management of PDPH, including the indications and contraindications for blood patching.*

Following total hip replacement and prolonged bed rest, there is an appreciable risk of deep venous thrombosis development, with subsequent risk of pulmonary embolism.

- **Question 7:** *What measures might be taken to minimise such a risk?*

FURTHER READING

Buckley N. Regional vs. general anaesthesia in orthopaedics. Can J Anaes 1993;
    40: R104–R108
Reilly C S. Regional anaesthesia and myocardial ischaemia (editorial). Br J Anaes 1993;
    71: 467–468
Reid J A, Thorburn J. Headache after spinal anaesthesia. (editorial). Br J Anaes 1991;
    67: 674–677
Reynolds F. Dural puncture and headache. (editorial). BMJ 1993; 306(8): 874–876
Jarvis A P, Creenawalt J W, Fragaeus L. Intravenous caffeine for post-dural puncture
    headache. Anes and Analg 1986; 65: 316–317
Prins I, Hirsh J. A comparison of general anesthesia and regional anesthesia as a risk factor
    for deep venous thrombosis following hip surgery: a critical review. Thrombosis and
    Haemostasis 1990; 64: 497–500
Carrie L E S. Post-dural puncture headache and extradural blood patch. (editorial).
    Br J Anaes 1993; 179–181

23 Rheumatoid arthritis

A 52-year-old male patient was admitted for elective right knee replacement. The patient had suffered from severe rheumatoid arthritis for 25 years and was severely incapacitated, requiring the use of a wheel chair to aid mobility. In addition to his rheumatoid arthritis he had experienced several episodes of sudden collapse in the last year which had been diagnosed as transient ischaemic attacks.

Current medication consisted of aspirin, penicillamine, ranitidine, gaviscon liquid p.r.n. and prednisolone. On examination the patient spoke with a hoarse voice, had trunkal obesity with marked cushingoid features and wore a soft surgical collar. His skin was thin with numerous striae over the abdomen. Suitable veins for cannulation were virtually non-existent. Bilateral ulnar deviation at the metacarpal phalangeal joints of the hands was pronounced and large effusions were present on both knees. Investigations included chest radiograph which was reported to show minimal bilateral pleural effusions and a minor degree of cardiomegaly. Cervical spine X-ray revealed a severe degree of atlanto-axial subluxation. A raised urea (15.8 mmol/l) and creatinine (198 mmol/l) were noted but electrolytes were normal. Haematological investigation showed a normochromic microcytic film with Hb 9.5 g/l, platelets 90 and a WBC $6.8 \times 10^9/l$. Urinalysis showed a +++ degree of proteinuria. Small voltage QRS complexes were seen on the ECG together with left axis deviation and left anterior hemiblock. The patient was keen to have the operation under an epidural anaesthetic after having had a discussion with another patient on the ward. After considerable discussion with the patient regarding the merits of regional and general anaesthesia in his particular case, it was decided to perform the operation under epidural with sedation. The patient was given temazepam as premedication 1 hour prior to surgery. With considerable difficulty venous access was eventually established by cut-down onto the large saphenous vein on the left leg at the ankle. Access to the epidural space was obtained with the patient in the left lateral position at the third lumbar interspace and a test dose of lignocaine administered. There were no signs of spinal nerve block 5 minutes later and bupivacaine was given. This produced a block to T10 and after sedation with increments of midazolam and the administration of oxygen via a Hudson mask, surgery commenced.

The arterial pressure decreased from 135/66 mmHg to 84/45 mmHg within the next 15 minutes. This hypotension was corrected using 500 mls of 0.9% saline solution and increments of methoxamine. Shortly after the last increment was administered, the patient developed complete heart block which reverted back to sinus rhythm with the administration of isoprenaline. The operation continued without further complication and the patient was transferred to the recovery room following the procedure. Over the following 4 hours blood loss from the drains was substantial and 5 units of red cell concentrate were transfused. The patient needed to go back to theatre for exploration of the wound and careful haemostasis was secured. The epidural catheter was topped up to provide suitable operating conditions for this exploratory operation. Postoperative analgesia was provided on the general ward by an epidural infusion of bupivacaine and fentanyl. This infusion continued for 48 hours.

The ward staff noted that the patient developed purpura and quite severe blistering of the skin where the ECG electrodes and the tape securing the epidural catheter had been. These improved over the next few weeks and the patient made an otherwise satisfactory recovery with physiotherapy and rehabilitation exercises.

DISCUSSION POINTS

The pre-operative assessment and investigations described in this case history are typical of any number of patients with rheumatoid disease presenting for orthopaedic operations. There are, however, certain features of this case that suggest the possibility of the additional diagnosis of amyloid disease.

- **Question 1:** *Discuss these and other features of the disease and how patients with this condition should be managed by the anaesthetist.*

Rheumatoid arthritis classically presents as a symmetrical involvement of the small and medium joints. Except for the upper cervical spine, the spine and sacroiliac joints are usually spared.

- **Question 2:** *Discuss the assessment of the cervical spine in the patient with rheumatoid arthritis and outline the airway management in such a patient.*

Central neural blockade using either epidural or spinal techniques is controversial when the patient is receiving therapy with aspirin and/or low molecular weight heparin, for fear of spinal haematoma formation leading to paralysis.

- *Question 3:* *Enlarge upon this controversial issue and assess the evidence for supporting the continued use of spinal and epidurals in patients on these drugs.*

- *Question 4:* *Describe the cardinal symptoms of a spinal haematoma that anaesthetists and attending physicians should be alert to.*

- *Question 5:* *Critically comment on the choice of technique for this patient, especially in the light of the increased tendency that patients with amyloid disease have for bleeding despite normal coagulation results.*

- *Question 6:* *Discuss in general terms the approach the anaesthetist should take when assessing a patient with rheumatoid disease for surgery.*

Many patients undergoing surgery using regional anaesthetic techniques find lying in one position for prolonged periods uncomfortable and understandably require sedation. Patients with rheumatoid disease often have fixed limb deformities and delicate skin.

- *Question 7:* *Describe the requirements for the safe positioning of these patients on the operating table whilst still providing the surgeon and anaesthetist with access.*

FURTHER READING

Skues M A, Welchew E A. Anaesthesia for rheumatoid arthritis. (review). Anaesthesia 1993; 48: 989–97

Macarthur A, Kleiman S. Rheumatoid cervical joint disease – a challenge to the anaesthetist. Can J Anaes 1993; 40: 154–159

Welch D B. Anaesthesia and amyloidosis. (case report and discussion). Anaesthesia 1982; 37: 63–6

Macdonald R. Aspirin and extradural blocks (editorial). Br J Anaes 1991; 66: 1–3

Wildsmith J A W, McClure J H. Anticoagulant drugs and central neural blockade. (editorial). Anaesthesia 1991; 46: 613–14

Modig J. Spinal or epidural anaesthesia with low molecular weight heparin for thromboprophylaxis requires careful postoperative neurological observation. (editorial). Acta Anaesthesiol Scand 1992; 36: 603–4

Berqvist D, Linblad B, Matzsch T. Low molecular weight heparin for thromboprophylaxis and epidural/spinal anaesthesia – Is there a risk? (review). Acta Anaesthesiol Scand 1992; 36: 605–9

24

Brachial plexus block

A healthy 55-year-old man who suffered from Dupuytren's contractures affecting the palm and index and middle fingers of his right hand wished to remain awake during surgery.

Pre-operative assessment revealed that he was of slim build, a smoker and nervous about the prospect of a general anaesthetic. He drank socially but denied excessive alcohol consumption. There were no other significant findings. The surgeon anticipated the procedure would last approximately 2 hours and would require the use of a tourniquet. The technique of supraclavicular brachial plexus block was explained and the importance of reporting paraesthesiae was emphasised. Temazepam was prescribed for premedication.

On arrival in the anaesthetic room he appeared slightly anxious. Basic monitoring was established and intravenous access was established in the left arm. He was positioned with his head turned to the left.

The midpoint of his clavicle was marked and a weal raised on the skin about 1 cm above this point with lignocaine. A regional block needle was advanced backwards, inwards and downwards to a depth of about 3.5 cm, and at this point the patient suddenly moved and started to cough violently. The needle was immediately withdrawn and the patient settled but still coughed occasionally. Once a little more settled, however, he complained of a dull ache in the upper part of his chest on the affected side. Examination revealed distant breath sounds and a tympanic percussion note. A pneumothorax occupying about 25% of the affected lung field was confirmed on erect chest X-ray and the procedure was abandoned. The patient's symptoms settled with simple analgesia, and as there was no respiratory distress it was decided not to place a chest drain. The pneumothorax resorbed over 48 hours and his surgery was carried out under general anaesthesia the following week.

DISCUSSION POINTS

- *Question 1:* *There are a number of approaches to the brachial plexus. Describe these approaches and discuss the advantages and disadvantages of each. Do you think that the approach used in this case was the most appropriate?*

- **Question 2:** *There are a variety of methods of ensuring that the tip of the needle is in the correct position before injection. Can you discuss the advantages and disadvantages of these?*

- **Question 3:** *Intravascular injection of local anaesthetic is a potential complication of this technique. What are the signs and symptoms of this?*

- **Question 4:** *What factors influence the development of local anaesthetic toxicity when large volumes of local anaesthetic are used?*

- **Question 5:** *Neurological damage may result from regional anaesthesia. What would you tell the patient about this?*

The disadvantages of this particular technique are related to the proximity of important anatomical structures to the area where the needle is placed. Of particular importance is the dome of pleura which lies medial to the first rib: if this is punctured a pneumothorax results. The incidence of this complication is quoted at 0.5% to 6% and diminishes with experience.

- *Question 6:* *Do you think the decision not to drain the pneumothorax was correct?*

- *Question 7:* *What features of a pneumothorax would persuade you to place a chest drain?*

FURTHER READING

Hickey R, Ramamurthy S. Brachial plexus block. Current Opinion in Anes 1993; 6: 823–829

Wildsmith J A W, Armitage E eds. Regional anaesthesia. 2nd ed. Edinburgh: Churchill Livingstone, 1993

Brown D L, Cahil D R, Bridenbaugh D L. Supraclavicular nerve block: Anatomic analysis of a method to prevent pneumothorax. Anesthesia and Analgesia 1993; 76: 530–534

Chambers W A. Peripheral nerve damage and regional anaesthesia. (editorial). Br J Anaes 1992; 69: 429–430

Moore D C, Mulroy M S & Thompson G E. Peripheral nerve damage and regional anaesthesia. (editorial). Br J Anaes 1994; 435–436

25

Carcinoid

A 41-year-old woman was admitted to the medical ward for investigation following an episode of haemoptysis. A chest X-ray organised by her GP demonstrated a 2 cm lesion in the left lower lobe of lung. She admitted to having smoked 15 cigarettes a day for the last 20 years, but had cut this down to 5 per day since seeing her GP. Systematic enquiry revealed a 'smoker's cough' and a history of slight weight loss. She volunteered she had slept badly over the last two weeks, which she attributed to worry. On examination she was noted to be anxious and to weigh 57 kg but there were no other positive findings. Routine investigations included full blood count, urea and electrolytes liver function tests and pulmonary function tests. The results of these were unremarkable.

She was scheduled for bronchoscopy the next morning. At the pre-operative visit that evening the anaesthetist explained the sequence of events for the next day. When asked if she had any queries, she expressed anxiety about the result of the bronchoscopy but was not concerned about the anaesthetic itself. Premedication with temazepam orally was prescribed.

On arrival in the anaesthetic room basic monitoring was established. Anaesthesia was induced with propofol and alfentanil and maintained with isoflurane and 50% nitrous oxide in oxygen. Suxamethonium was given for muscle relaxation and a size 8.5 cuffed orotracheal tube was placed without difficulty. Bronchoscopy revealed a lesion in the left lower lobe. When biopsied the lesion bled profusely but after some time this settled. Anaesthesia was discontinued and once spontaneous respiration had returned, the patient was extubated after suctioning of the respiratory passages.

In recovery room she was alert, frequently coughed blood-stained sputum and complained of a sore throat. She was cardiovascularly stable and the coughing gradually reduced. Fifty minutes later, when the coughing had settled to a significant degree, she returned to the ward.

Histology of the biopsy revealed adenomatous tissue. The patient was informed of the result and after discussion was scheduled for a left thoracotomy with the intention of carrying out a left thoracotomy 3 days later.

DISCUSSION POINTS

Histology and friability of the tumour at biopsy suggested that carcinoid tumour was a possibility in this case, although carcinoid tumours form less than 1% of bronchial tumours. Associated with carcinoid tumours is the carcinoid syndrome. Although less than 25% of patients with a carcinoid tumour develop the syndrome, it has important implications for the anaesthetic management.

- **Question 1:** *What conditions are necessary for the development of the carcinoid syndrome and what symptoms might the patient have experienced had she developed this syndrome?*

Some investigations were performed in this patient prior to bronchoscopy: full blood count, urea and electrolytes, liver function tests, blood sugar and chest X-ray. Additional investigations prior to thoracotomy will include CT scan of lung, ultrasound of liver, bone scan, pulmonary function tests and ECG.

- **Question 2:** *What abnormalities might you expect in a patient with carcinoid syndrome?*

The carcinoid syndrome results from episodic release of mediators capable of influencing vascular, bronchial and gastrointestinal smooth muscle. Principally serotonin and bradykinin are involved, but more than 20 substances – including peptide hormones such as gastrin, ACTH, growth hormone, calcitonin, insulin and glucagon – are known to be produced by carcinoid tumours.

- **Question 3:** *Discuss the problems this might present during anaesthesia, how you would monitor the patient, and what anaesthetic technique you could use to minimise the problems.*

• **Question 4:** *Are there any drugs you can use to control the syndrome during anaesthesia?*

In the past, rigid bronchoscopy might have been performed for the pre-operative location of tumours and assessment of carinal and bronchial rigidity. However, with improvement of imaging techniques (e.g. CT scan) its use is now primarily for the removal of foreign bodies.

• **Question 5:** *What are the options for ventilating a patient during a rigid bronchoscopy?*

Haemorrhage may be a complication of biopsy during rigid or flexible bronchoscopy.

• **Question 6:** *How might this be managed?*

• **Question 7:** *What other complications might arise and how might these be treated?*

FURTHER READING

Batchelor A M, Conacher I D. Anaphylactoid or carcinoid? Br J Anaes 1992; 69: 325–7

Ricci C, Patresi I, Massa R, Bendeti-Valenti F. Carcinoid syndrome in bronchial adenoma. Am J Surg 1973; 126: 671–7

Mason R A, Steane P A. Carcinoid syndrome: its relevance to the anaesthetist. Anaesthesia 1976; 31: 228–242

Roy R C, Carter R F, Wright P D. Somatostatin, anaesthesia, and the carcinoid syndrome. Anaesthesia 1987; 42: 627–32

Veall G R Q, Peacock J E, Bax N D S, Reilly C S. Review of the anaesthetic management of 21 patients undergoing laparotomy for carcinoid syndrome. Br J Anaes 1994; 72: 335–341

26 Mediastinal mass

A 26-year-old male presented with a history of shortness of breath on exertion, worsening over the last 6 weeks. It was associated with slight wheeze. He also complained of difficulty in breathing when lying flat, and a chronic non-productive cough. Chest X-ray showed a large mediastinal mass (Fig. 26.1) and CT scan confirmed the presence of an anterior mediastinal mass with some compression of the distal trachea. He was referred for mediastinoscopy for tissue diagnosis, prior to definitive treatment.

Flow volume loops performed in the supine and upright positions suggested marked intra-thoracic airway obstruction when supine. Other than this, his general health was good and at the pre-operative visit he seemed relaxed, but refused to have any procedures undertaken unless he was fully anaesthetised.

The patient was premedicated with temazepam orally. He arrived in the anaesthetic room supine but with the trolley inclined to 45°. He denied any difficulty in breathing and appeared calm with an oxygen saturation of 98% breathing air. Following 3 minutes pre-oxygenation, alfentanil was administered and then anaesthesia was induced with propofol which was titrated until there was loss of eyelash reflex. Blood pressure and heart rate were stable but the airway became obstructed. Attempts to inflate the lungs by mask were unsuccessful. Tracheal intubation was carried out easily, but still inflation of the lungs was impossible. The tube was removed and the thoracic surgeon, who had been standing by, was asked to

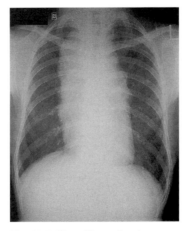

Fig. 26.1 Chest X-ray showing mediastinal lymphadenopathy

pass a rigid bronchoscope. This was achieved easily following a further dose of propofol. Compression of the distal trachea was confirmed; however the rigid scope could be passed beyond the compression to reveal distorted but patent bronchi distal to the carina. The lungs could then easily be inflated by Venturi ventilation. In view of the ease of ventilation it was decided to leave the rigid bronchoscope in situ. The operation proceeded uneventfully, anaesthesia being maintained with a propofol infusion and muscle relaxation provided with atracurium. At the end of the procedure the patient was turned onto his left side and the rigid bronchoscope was removed. In this position it proved relatively easy to ventilate the lungs. Muscle relaxation was reversed with neostigmine and glycopyrrolate and spontaneous ventilation was achieved within a few minutes. Thereafter the recovery from this procedure was uneventful.

DISCUSSION POINTS

Patients with symptomatic anterior mediastinal masses are potentially at grave risk during induction of anaesthesia. These risks can be minimised by:

- The use of local anaesthesia both for examination and subsequent intubation of the airway.
- The maintenance of spontaneous ventilation.
- The presence of staff experienced in the use of a rigid bronchoscope.

- *Question 1: Can you comment on each of these points?*

- *Question 2: Discuss the investigation and clinical assessment of these patients.*

Despite a clear airway some of these patients may suffer cardiovascular collapse during induction of anaesthesia.

● **Question 3:** *What are the mechanisms which produce this and how might they be managed?*

FURTHER READING

Nean G G, Weingarten A E, Abramowitz R M, Kussens L G, Absons A L, Lassner W. The anaesthetic management of the patient with anterior mediastinal mass. Anesthesiology 1984; 60: 144–7

Ferrari L R, Bedford R F. General anaesthesia prior to treatment of anterior mediastinal masses in paediatric cancer patients. Anesthesiology 1990; 72: 991–5

Yoker D, Clark R, Coreler L. Fibreoptic endobronchial intubation for resection of an anterior mediastinal mass. Anesthesiology 1989; 70: 144–6

Joivson D, Hurst T, Cujec B, Mayers I. Cardiopulmonary effects of an anterior mediastinal mass in dogs anaesthetised with halothane. Anesthesiology 1991; 70: 725–36

Goth J W W, Macrae D J. 'Thoracic anaesthetic problems' In: Balliere's Clinical Anaesthesiology. March 1987; 1: 107–31

27 Thymectomy

A 17-year-old girl with myasthenia gravis was scheduled for elective trans-sternal thymectomy. She had presented to the neurologists with difficulty in swallowing 3 months previously. The diagnosis had been made and she had been commenced on pyridostigmine orally 5 times a day which had controlled her symptoms except when she awoke in the morning. She had no significant past medical history, and systematic enquiry and physical examination were unremarkable. Chest X-ray was normal, as were her haemoglobin and full blood count, and urea and electrolytes. Pulmonary function tests were also performed and were within normal limits. Pyridostigmine was continued up to the time of surgery which was scheduled for one hour after the last dose. No pre-medication was given. Routine monitoring including a radial arterial line was established and anaesthesia induced with fentanyl, propofol and droperidol. After ventilation by face mask with 50% nitrous oxide in oxygen, the trachea was intubated without difficulty. Anaesthesia was maintained with 66% nitrous oxide in oxygen and an intravenous propofol infusion which was adjusted to maintain stable cardiovascular parameters.

Anaesthesia and surgery proceeded uneventfully and the operation was completed in 2 hours. As the skin was being sutured the propofol was discontinued and pyridostigmine and glycopyrrolate administered intravenously. The patient awoke 5 minutes after the completion of the surgery, ventilation and coughing were judged to be adequate and she was extubated. At this time the response of the adductor pollicis to train-of-four stimulation of the ulnar nerve was normal.

Postoperative analgesia consisted of a diclofenac suppository daily for 3 days and morphine via a patient controlled analgesia system. She was able to take her oral pyridostigmine normally 2 hours after surgery was completed and this was continued into the postoperative period which was uneventful.

DISCUSSION POINTS

- *Question 1:* Can you describe the physiological defect in myasthenia gravis and the response of these patients to neuromuscular blocking drugs?

• **Question 2:** *What postoperative complications are likely in a myasthenic patient?*

Thymectomy is now being offered much earlier in the myasthenia gravis disease process than it was in the past, and the need for postoperative ventilation has diminished. It is obviously essential that the facilities for this are available even if minor surgery is undertaken in myasthenics. The bio-availability of pyridostigmine is only 3–8% when administered orally due to poor absorption from the gastro-intestinal tract. The intravenous dose is obviously much less.

• **Question 3:** *What are the potential dangers of giving an excessive dose of the anti-cholinesterase?*

Non-depolarising neuromuscular blockade has been successfully used during thymectomy, particularly with vecuronium and atracurium.

• **Question 4:** *If you chose this technique, what dosage would you use and how would you ensure complete reversal?*

Transcervical thymectomy is said to incur less postoperative respiratory complications than when the operation is carried out through the trans-sternal route.

● **Question 5:** *Why, therefore, is the trans-sternal technique usually preferred?*

● **Question 6:** *What are the advantages of propofol for this procedure in this type of patient over the volatile anaesthetic agents?*

FURTHER READING

Redfern N, McQuillan P J, Conacher I D, Pearson D T. Anaesthesia for trans-sternal thymectomy in myasthenia gravis. Ann RCSE 1987; 69: 289–292

Barraka A, TabbDush Z. Neuromuscular response to succinylcholine vecuronium sequence in three myasthenic patients undergoing thymectomy. Anes Analg 1991; 72: 827–830

Burgess F, Wilkosky B. Thoracic epidural anaesthesia for trans-sternal thymectomy in myasthenia gravis. Anes Analg 1989; 69: 529–31

Rowbottom S J. Isoflurane for thymectomy in myasthenia gravis. Anaesth Intensive Care 1989; 17: 444–447

28 Thoracotomy

A 26-year-old female patient had a soft tissue sarcoma removed from her leg under a combination of general and epidural anaesthesia. Despite a self-confessed needle phobia and low pain threshold postoperatively, she had no major peri-operative problems. She remained well for 2 years, but routine chest X-ray revealed a discrete solitary lesion in her left lung, thought to be a secondary deposit (Fig. 28.1). Following investigation she presented for left lower lobectomy. Her general health was good, but she was extremely anxious about the prospect of surgery, and in particular, her ability to cope with pain.

The pre-operative course was difficult, and despite full explanation of the various options available and reassurance about the likely effects of analgesic regimes, she remained tense and tearful. The night before surgery lorazepam was given and she slept well. A further dose was given the following morning and EMLA cream applied to both hands. On arrival in the anaesthetic room she was awake but appeared relaxed, and intravenous access was established without incident. It was planned to site a thoracic epidural catheter before induction of anaesthesia, but despite a bolus of midazolam she became agitated as her back was being prepared. Catheter placement was deferred, and induction of anaesthesia and intubation took place without further incident. A thoracic epidural

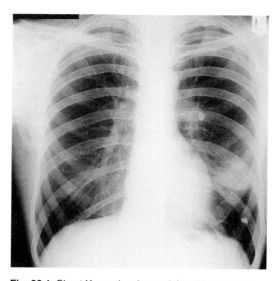

Fig. 28.1 Chest X-ray showing peripheral lung lesion

catheter was placed at the T5-6 level and thereafter anaesthesia and surgery proceeded uneventfully. Prior to and during surgery she received bupivacaine via the epidural catheter and alfentanil and morphine intravenously.

In the recovery room she was initially drowsy. An infusion of bupivacaine was commenced via the epidural catheter. Fifteen minutes later she started to complain of severe right shoulder pain and was given morphine intravenously and diclofenac per rectum. Her pain decreased and within 30 minutes she was virtually pain-free and stable. During this time a patient controlled analgesia system (PCA) was prepared and she was reminded of how and when to use the pump. The syringe contained morphine and droperidol and a background infusion was not used.

She remained comfortable in the high-dependency unit and for the first 8 hours did not use the PCA. However later that evening she started to complain of pain from the lower chest drain site, and although use of the PCA was encouraged she remained uncomfortable.

The anaesthetist was contacted but was unable to attend immediately and suggested a further bolus of morphine. This was titrated to effect by the House Officer, and thereafter she continued to use the PCA successfully for a further 2 hours. At this time she was seen by the anaesthetist, who confirmed regression of the initial epidural block and gave a further bolus dose of bupivacaine. The epidural was removed 20 hours later just prior to a dose of heparin, and she remained comfortable over the next 24 hours, with her pain controlled by morphine and diclofenac.

DISCUSSION POINTS

Many anaesthetists favour a combined pharmacological approach to the relief of pain after thoracotomy, using local anaesthetics, opioids and non steroidal anti-inflammatory drugs.

- *Question 1:* *Can you describe the options for delivery of local anaesthetic agents e.g. epidural, intercostal, paravertebral, intrapleural, and what the particular advantages and disadvantages are for each technique?*

Shoulder tip pain is common after thoracotomy.

• **Question 2:** *What is the aetiology, and how can it be managed?*

The addition of opioids to the epidural space either alone or in combination with local anaesthetics is popular.

• **Question 3:** *Which drugs are commonly used and why?*

• **Question 4:** *What are the potential benefits and drawbacks of each drug?*

This case highlights problems in providing good pain relief after thoracotomy, and in particular those associated with block regression and sub-therapeutic blood levels of analgesic agents.

• **Question 5:** *How can these practical points be addressed?*

- **Question 6:** *Can you comment on the desirability or otherwise of siting a thoracic epidural in an awake patient?*

- **Question 7:** *Can you discuss the use of regional techniques in the presence of drugs which can affect coagulation?*

FURTHER READING

Conacher I D. Pain relief after thoracotomy. Br J Anaes 1990; 65: 806–812

O'Connor C J. Thoracic epidural anaesthesia: physiological effects and clinical applications. J Cardiothoracic and Vascular Anaes 1993; 7: 595–609

Grant R, Dolman J F, Harper J A, Adrian White S, Parsos D G, Evans K G, Merrick C P. Patient controlled lumbar epidural fentanyl compared with patient controlled intravenous fentanyl for post-thoracotomy pain. Can J Anaes 1992; 39: 214–219

Chan V W S, Chung F, Cheng D C H, Seyonne C, Chang A, Kirby T J. Analgesic and pulmonary effects of continuous intercostal nerve block following thoracotomy. Can J Anaes 1991; 38: 733–9

Sabananthan S, Mearns A J, Bickford Smith P I, Grisford R G, Bibby S R, Najid M R. Efficacy of continuous extra-pleural intercostal nerve block on post thoracotomy pain and pulmonary mechanics. Br J Surg 1990; 77: 221–5

Burgess F W, Anderson D M, Colonna D, Shorov M J, Cavanough D G. Ipsilateral shoulder pain following thoracic surgery. Anaesthesiology 1993; 78: 365–8. And correspondence in Anaesthesiology 1993; 79: 193

Bromage P R. The control of post-thoracotomy pain (correspondence). Reply: Vaughan R S, Gough J D. Anaesthesia 1989; 44: 445–446

Wildsmith J A W, McClure J H. Anticoagulant drugs and central nerve blockade (editorial). Anaesthesia 1991; 46: 613–614

Matthews P J, Govenden V. Comparison of continuous paravertebral and extradural infusion of bupivacaine for pain relief after thoracotomy. Br J Anaes 1989; 62: 204–205

29 Aortic surgery

An 18-year-old male was involved in a road traffic accident, sustaining fractures of the left femur, ankle, sternum and multiple abrasions. He had been knocked out at the scene but on admission was awake with a Glasgow Coma Scale of 14. He was resuscitated with 2 l of starch solution and 2 units packed cells and on reviewing his X-rays was noted to have a widened mediastinum (Fig. 29.1). A cardiothoracic opinion was sought and digital subtraction angiography (Fig. 29.2) confirmed an aortic tear distal to the origin of the left subclavian artery.

On arrival in the anaesthetic room, a 20 G cannula was placed in the right radial artery and anaesthesia was induced with fentanyl and midazolam. A 39 FG left-sided endobronchial double-lumen tube was placed and the position confirmed by fibre-optic bronchoscopy. An 8 FG cannula was placed in the left internal jugular vein alongside a triple-lumen catheter. After turning to the right lateral position, tube position was again verified with the bronchoscope. Surgery proceeded and at this stage, no effort was made to maintain normal body temperature.

Following collapse of the left lung, good exposure of the aorta was achieved and just prior to application of the aortic clamp, thiopentone was given intravenously and a glyceryl trinitrate (GTN) infusion was commenced. As the blood pressure fell, the aortic clamp was applied

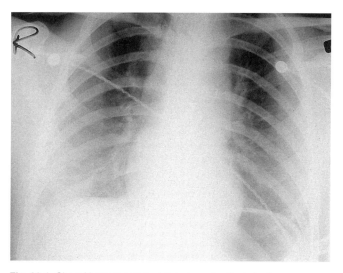

Fig. 29.1 Chest X-ray showing widened mediastinal shadow

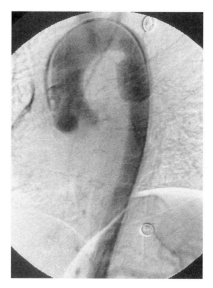

Fig. 29.2 Angiogram confirming leakage from the aorta

producing a rise in systolic pressure of 80 mmHg. This was controlled with further bolus doses of GTN and the rapid venesection of 500 ml of blood via the 8 FG cannula into a standard blood collection bag. Operative repair of the aortic tear took 45 minutes, during which time the patient remained stable with a core temperature of 35°C. The aortic clamp was released gradually and the 500 ml of autologous blood and 1200 ml of plasma were infused rapidly via blood warmers. The blood pressure was restored to post-induction level with bolus doses of phenylephrine and an infusion of adrenaline. As the suture line was inspected, metabolic acidosis and anaemia were corrected but the whole operative site appeared oozy. Four units of fresh frozen plasma and 6 units of platelets were given during closure of the chest. He was admitted to ITU for elective ventilation. Blood loss from the drains eventually subsided and the following morning he was extubated, having remained haemodynamically stable overnight. On examination he was found to have a paraparesis, but within 5 days normal sensation had returned to both legs.

DISCUSSION POINTS

Anaesthesia for surgery of the descending thoracic aorta presents one of the greatest challenges for the anaesthetist, and cases are usually referred to specialist centres. However, some general principles are relevant.
Good access to the aorta is essential in order to reduce cross-clamp time and this requires one lung anaesthesia.

- **Question 1:** *Can you describe the blood supply to the spinal cord?*

- **Question 2:** *What particular aspects of the anatomy make the cord particularly vulnerable during aortic clamping in the thoracic region?*

- **Question 3:** *Can you describe the haemodynamic consequences of clamping the aorta at this level? How may this be managed?*

Paraplegia is the most feared complication of this type of surgery.

- **Question 4:** *What is the incidence of this complication and how may it be minimised? (It may be easier to consider this under the headings Flow, Pressure, Drugs, Temperature).*

Evoked potentials have been suggested as a means of early detection of conduction disturbance along nerve pathways.

- ***Question 5:*** *What are evoked potentials, how are they measured and how good are they in predicting a poor outcome?*

Clotting factors were given empirically to this patient.

- ***Question 6:*** *How should clotting disturbances occurring during surgery be managed?*

FURTHER READING

Spargo P M, Crosse M M. Anaesthetic problems in cross-clamping of the thoracic aorta. Ann RCSE 1988; 70: 64–68

Sheraq S A. Anaesthesia for thoracic aortic aneurysms. Current Opinion in Anaesthesiology 1992; 5: 62–67

Sheraq S A, Svensson C G. Paraplegia following aortic surgery. J Cardiothoracic and Vascular Anaes 1993; 7: 81–84

Mutch W A C, Thomson I R, Teskey J M, Thiesson D, Rosenbloom M. Phlebotomy reverses the haemodynamic consequences of thoracic aortic cross-clamping: relationships between central venous pressure and cerebrospinal fluid pressure. Anaesthesiology 1991; 74: 320–324

Drenger B, Parker S, McPherson R, North R, Melville Williams G, Reitz B A, Beattie C. Spinal cord stimulation evoked potentials during thoracoabdominal aortic aneurysm surgery. Anaesthesiology 1992; 76: 689–695

Donaldson M D J, Seaman M J, Park G R. Massive blood transfusion. Br J Anaes 1992; 69: 621–630

A 52-year-old farmer presented for the first stage of maxillofacial reconstruction following a failed suicide attempt 2 days previously. He had placed the barrel of a twelve-bore shotgun under his chin, but while pulling the trigger the barrel had deflected so the contents of the cartridge exited through his right cheek. Widespread damage of the soft tissues and multiple fractures of the mandible and right maxilla resulted (Fig. 30.1). He was fully orientated and CNS observations had been normal since admission. There was obvious severe damage to the soft tissues of the floor of the mouth, and it was assumed within, but this could not be assessed due to inability to open the mouth. Congealed blood was caked around the mouth and nostrils and all these areas bled to touch. X-rays showed extensive bony damage, with bone fragments and teeth in the mouth and anterior pharynx. There was no radiological evidence of inhaled foreign material. Past medical history, physical examination and investigations were otherwise unremarkable.

As long-term tracheostomy was necessary for the multi-stage reconstruction, and in light of the severe facial damage, it was decided – in consultation with the maxillo-facial surgeon – that this procedure be carried out under local anaesthesia prior to the induction of general anaesthesia. The tracheostomy was carried out uneventfully with local infiltra-

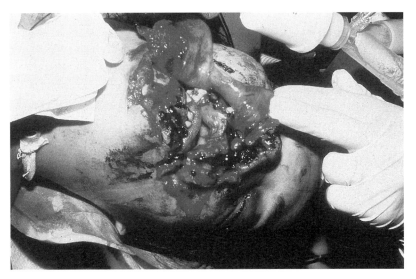

Fig. 30.1

tion of lignocaine. Once the correct position of the tracheostomy tube was confirmed, general anaesthesia was induced conventionally and surgery proceeded uneventfully.

DISCUSSION POINTS

- *Question 1:* Do you think other methods of establishing a clear airway, such as fibre-optic laryngoscopy and intubation, cricothyrotomy or percutaneous tracheostomy, might have had a place in the management of this patient?

Anatomy of this patient's airway was considerably distorted by his injury, although he could maintain it while conscious.

- *Question 2:* Discuss the dangers of inducing general anaesthesia in this type of patient without first ensuring a secure airway.

This patient had a normal level of consciousness throughout.

- *Question 3:* Had he sustained a significant head injury and required control of the airway urgently, how would you proceed?

• **Question 4:** *Would the mechanism of injury lead you to suspect any other injuries?*

Assessment of the airway and potential problems with airway maintenance are an essential part of any anaesthetic pre-operative assessment. Only then can appropriate planning take place. Many different methods have been described to aid this assessment.

• **Question 5:** *Are any of these fail-safe?*

• **Question 6:** *Which methods do you use at the bedside?*

• **Question 7:** *Outline the equipment you would require if setting up a difficult intubation trolley for your theatre.*

FURTHER READING

Griggs W, Myburgh I, Worthley L. Urgent airway access – an indication for percutaneous tracheostomy? Anaesth Intensive Care 1991; 19: 586–587
Bodenham A R. Percutaneous dilational tracheostomy: completing the anaesthetists range of airway techniques. Anaesthesia 1993; 48: 101–102

Colby M, Vaughan R S. Recognition and management of difficult airway problems. Br J Anaes 1992; 86(1): 90–97

King T A, Adams A P. Failed tracheal intubation. Br J Anaes 1990; 65: 400–414

Wilson M E. Predicting difficult intubation. Br J Anaes 1993; 71: 333–334

Frerk C M. Predicting difficult intubation. Anaesthesia 1991; 46: 1005–1008

Salvino C K, Dries D, Gamelli R, Murphy-Macabobby M, Marshall W. Emergency cricothyroidotomy in trauma victims. J Trauma 1993; 34: 503–505

31 Aeromedical transport

The anaesthetist on call at a remote district general hospital was asked by the physicians to see a 50-year-old woman admitted during the night with headache and reduced level of consciousness. It was planned to transfer her to the nearest neurosurgical unit for urgent investigation and management as her condition had deteriorated significantly since admission. In view of the reduced level of consciousness, it was felt she should be accompanied by an anaesthetist during the transfer, and due to the distance to the neurosurgical centre and the rapid deterioration in condition, air transfer by helicopter was planned.

A limited history was available. She was known to have complained of morning headaches over the last 2 weeks. On the night prior to admission she noticed blurring of vision, complained of nausea and vomited several times. She smoked 20 cigarettes per day, but otherwise past medical history was unremarkable. On examination at admission her Glasgow Coma Scale (GCS) was 12 (E3, M5, V4) and there was thought to be bilateral papilloedema. Chest X-ray and ECG were normal, as were the admission blood investigations (full blood count and urea and electrolytes). The presumptive diagnosis was of an intracranial space-occupying lesion of unknown origin, and in light of signs of raised intracranial pressure (ICP), she was commenced on dexamethasone.

When the anaesthetist assessed her, the GCS was 8 (E2, M3, V2). The nurse reported that she did not appear to be breathing as well as before. An infusion of mannitol was in progress, and she had just been catheterised. In view of the reduced level of consciousness, and the impending transfer, the anaesthetist decided to intubate and ventilate the patient. She was rapidly transferred to an anaesthetic room where basic monitoring was established and after 3 minutes pre-oxygenation, alfentanil, thiopentone and suxamethonium were administered intravenously. An oral-cuffed endotracheal tube was inserted and the patient was hyperventilated to produce an end tidal CO_2 of 3.5–4 kPa. Intravenous infusions of propofol and atracurium were started and she was transferred onto the helicopter stretcher system and wrapped in a space blanket. A portable ventilator was used. On arrival at the helipad she was transferred from the ambulance into the helicopter (Fig. 31.1) and monitoring of the ECG, pulse oximetry, non-invasive blood pressure and end tidal CO_2 were continued on battery-powered machines.

Flight time was just over one hour. Fifteen minutes into the flight the patient developed bradycardia and hypertension. Pupillary signs were

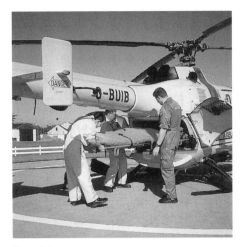

Fig. 31.1

unchanged. A further intravenous bolus of mannitol was given with intravenous frusemide. The cardiovascular signs seemed to stabilise over the next 20 minutes. Ten minutes from landing the S_pO_2 fell to 90%, the end tidal CO_2 rose and hypertension and tachycardia developed. The anaesthetist examined the patient and decided there was poor expansion of the left side of her chest. On auscultation there seemed to be diminished air entry on the left side. Cautiously the endotracheal tube was withdrawn 2 cm and air entry improved. The S_pO_2, end tidal CO_2, heart rate and blood pressure returned to previous levels.

The remainder of the flight was uneventful. Following a further short ambulance journey from the helipad to the neurosurgical intensive care unit, the patient was handed over to the neurosurgical receiving team.

DISCUSSION POINTS

Headache, especially in the morning, nausea and vomiting, with papilloedema are a classical presentation of raised ICP. Unilateral pupil changes may occur. Changes in level of consciousness and respiratory pattern are relatively late signs.

- *Question 1:* *How can ICP be measured?*

• **Question 2:** *What do you understand by the term 'intracranial compliance'?*

• **Question 3:** *Discuss the management of a patient with raised ICP.*

Aeromedical transport has many logistical and operational implications. Although helicopters can take off or land in very small areas and would therefore appear perfect for hospital to hospital transfer, in practice they may not be quite so ideal. Many of the civilian helicopters used for such transfers are small, and so although they fulfil the criteria for rapid transfer from A to B, they may not be suitable for intensive resuscitation and management en route. They tend to be noisy. Fixed-wing aircraft travel rapidly and are almost certainly more comfortable, but can only fly airport to airport.

Helicopter transport will be smoother and avoid the rapid acceleration – deceleration characteristics of land ambulance transfer, but may have other disadvantages for certain patients. Patient loading and unloading may have to be performed with care to avoid extremes of head-up or head-down position. Helicopters accelerate in a slightly 'nose'-down position and so patients with elevated ICP should fly 'feet first' wherever possible. However, in the small craft used for aeromedical evacuation in some parts of the UK, this would leave the patient's head and airway completely inaccessible (Fig. 31.1).

• **Question 4:** *What other advantages and disadvantages do they have over land transfer? Compare other advantages and disadvantages of fixed wing and rotor aeromedical transfer.*

● **Question 5:** *What monitoring would you want on these transfers and what problems might be associated with your choice?*

● **Question 6:** *Discuss the effects of altitude on a patient with respiratory problems.*

FURTHER READING

Harding R M, Mills F I. Aviation Medicine. 3rd ed. BMJ Publishing, 1993
Mulrooney P. Aeromedical patient transfer. Br J Hosp Med 1991; 45: 209–212
de Mello W F, Thompson M. The disadvantages of helicopter transfer (letter). Br J Hosp Med 1990; 43: 328
Working Party Report: Recommended standards for UK fixed-wing medical air transport systems and for patient management during transfer by fixed-wing aircraft. J Royal Soc Med 1992; 85: 767–71
Ravussin P. Neurological sedation and control of intracranial volume and pressure. Anaesthesia Rounds. Medicine Group (Education) Abington, England 1993

32 Extrication of a train crash victim

An emergency team consisting of an accident surgeon, a general surgeon, an orthopaedic surgeon and an anaesthetist with basic surgical instruments, dressings, antibiotics, intravenous fluids and intravenous analgesic and anaesthetic agents attended the site of the head-on collision of two passenger trains.

The driver of one train was found to be alive but trapped, his cab having collapsed on top of him on impact. He was conscious and coherent but having difficulty breathing and complained of severe pain in his legs. Only his right arm was accessible through a small opening which had been made in the wall dividing the cab from the passenger saloon. Through this gap he was given cyclimorph intramuscularly, the needle being passed through the sleeve of his jacket. A further 25 minutes passed before the dividing wall could be broken down and he was able to pass his right arm through. A strong radial pulse was identified, and a 14 G cannula was sited in the dorsum of the hand. A further dose of cyclimorph was given intravenously, and one litre of polygeline infused. The remainder of the partition was removed and it became apparent that the casualty was trapped between the wreckage of the front of the train which had collapsed on top of him, and the driver's chair behind. The chair was cut away, freeing his upper body from the wreckage; this resulted in an immediate improvement in his breathing, and oxygen could now be commenced through a Hudson-type mask and ECG monitoring was established. Both legs remained trapped some 18 inches above floor level in such a fashion that he was forced to adopt a semi-lateral position and several layers of padding were placed underneath his trunk. The fire-fighters continued their efforts to free the victim's legs, using heavy lifting and cutting equipment, and this caused severe pain. In the absence of a revealed head injury (GCS 15 and no sign of head trauma), and because the casualty's position prevented the easy passage of an endotracheal tube, ketamine was administered intravenously to provide analgesia during further attempts to free the legs. This resulted in loss of consciousness but without obvious detrimental effect on respiration. Further attempts by the fire-fighters resulted in freeing of the right leg, but it proved impossible to release the left leg.

Over 2 hours following the arrival of the emergency team, a further one litre of polygeline, one litre of normal saline and three units of group 0 Rh negative-packed cells were transfused. The patient was breathing spontaneously, but was unconscious, hypothermic, and no peripheral pulse was detectable. It appeared that there were no gross head, chest or abdominal injuries present, all trauma being limited to the lower limbs which were grossly deformed. The air temperature was falling and daylight would begin to fade in another hour's time. In view of the desperate situation, it was decided that the only possibility of saving this victim lay in amputation of the left foot. A further dose of ketamine was given, and because of the position of the trapped leg, it was necessary for the surgeon to work from outside the train standing on a ladder, and reaching into the driver's cab. Skin incision produced no response from the patient, and the foot was crudely amputated proximal to the ankle joint. The patient was then able to be pulled back into the passenger compartment where an area had been cleared of all unnecessary equipment and seating and a second surgeon applied a tourniquet to the leg and clipped obvious bleeding vessels. An attempt was made to intubate the patient but this proved impossible under the prevailing conditions. Tracheostomy was not considered appropriate as the patient had a patent airway, adequate respiration and this procedure would have delayed evacuation.

The patient was placed on a stretcher and carried across several tracks to an ambulance. He was then transferred to the receiving hospital accompanied by anaesthetist and surgeon. On arrival at the Accident and Emergency Department, further assessment and resuscitation were performed and the patient was taken to theatre for wound toilet and fixation of fractures followed by admission to ITU for postoperative IPPV. A coagulopathy developed and was treated with repeated transfusion of concentrated red cells, fresh-frozen plasma, cryoprecipitate and platelets. Renal function, gas exchange and cardiovascular function remained good and the patient was discharged from ITU after 24 hours.

DISCUSSION POINTS

This type of case represents a major challenge to the resourcefulness of anaesthetists. Most of us are unprepared for this sort of situation but must overcome our anxiety to apply the basic principles of resuscitation which have been learnt in a hospital environment. It is essential that all staff familiarise themselves in advance of an emergency with the equipment and drugs which will be available.

Ketamine was used to provide anaesthesia in this instance.

● *Question 1:* *Which features of this drug made it a suitable choice?*

• *Question 2: Describe the problems which may arise with its use.*

In this situation restricted access and space made the use of inhalational anaesthesia impossible.

• *Question 3: Describe the equipment necessary to provide inhalational anaesthesia in the field.*

This incident involved the management of one trapped victim, with four senior doctors at the scene, and a full emergency service team able to concentrate on his extrication. Decisions and management of this case were made giving full attention to the well-being of the victim, the safety of the rescue workers, environmental conditions and the need to complete the job of wreckage clearance. Contrast this with a multiple casualty situation, when the numbers of casualties stress the medical and rescue service resources such that treatment must be prioritised so victims with the most urgent needs receive the earliest definitive care; or the mass casualty situation when resources are so over-loaded that triage needs to direct resources to those with the greatest opportunity for survival.

In regard to these two situations:

• *Question 4: What are your treatment priorities for victims in the multiple casualty incident and in what order will you apply them?*

- **Question 5:** *How would you categorise victims in the mass casualty incident?*

- **Question 6:** *What are your treatment priorities at the scene in these two situations?*

- **Question 7:** *How will you communicate decisions and findings at the scene to ambulance personnel transferring victims and the definitive care centre receiving them?*

On arrival at hospital victims should again undergo triage and be reassigned their category, as a 20–30% error rate in the categories of field triage may be present.

- **Question 8:** *Who should be making triage decisions in the field and at the receiving centre? Should this always be medical staff?*

● ***Question 9:*** *How would you organise the hospital to receive accident victims from a multiple or mass situation? Which grades and types of personnel do you want in the different assessment and treatment areas?*

FURTHER READING

Restall J, Thomson M C, Johnston I G, Fenton T C. Anaesthesia in the field. Spontaneous ventilation – a new technique. Anaesthesia 1990; 45: 965–968

Wilson R J, Ridley S A. The use of propofol and alfentanil by infusion in military anaesthesia. Anaesthesia 1992; 47: 231–233

Martin T E. Resolving the casualty evacuation conflict. Injury 1993; 24: 514–516

Johnstone D J, Evans S C, Field R E, Booth S J. The Victoria bomb: a report from the Westminster Hospital. Injury 1993; 24: 5–9

Hodgetts T J. Lessons from the Musgrave Park Hospital bombing. Injury 1993; 24: 219–221

Nancekievill D G. On-site medical services at major incidents. Training still the black spot. BMJ 1992; 305: 726–727

33 Carotid artery surgery

A 65-year-old man presented to the neurology department with a recent history of transient ischaemic attacks affecting his right arm and vision. Three years previously he suffered an inferior myocardial infarction, from which he made an uncomplicated recovery. Other medical problems included hypertension for 2 years and non-insulin-dependant diabetes mellitus for 5 years. Systematic enquiry revealed occasional chest tightness after walking up the steep hill home in cold windy weather during the last 4 months. Current drug therapy consisted of metformin and nifedipine. He smoked 10 cigarettes per day.

On examination pulse rate was 60/min, and blood pressure 150/90 mmHg. Auscultation of the chest revealed no abnormality, but a left carotid bruit was heard. There was no neurological deficit. Chest X-ray, full blood count, urea and electrolytes were within normal limits and monitoring of blood sugar gave values of 9–14 mmol/l. Due to the recent history of chest tightness, an exercise ECG was performed. He completed 10 minutes of the standard Bruce protocol, stopping due to exhaustion. At this point there were no ischaemic changes on the ECG, no dysrhythmias, no fall in blood pressure and the patient had achieved 85% of maximal heart rate. No further investigation of his myocardial state was performed. Doppler ultrasound of his carotid arteries revealed an 80% stenosis of the left carotid artery, and CT scan of his head revealed no cerebral infarcts. In light of this severe degree of stenosis and symptoms, the patient was referred to the vascular surgeons and was scheduled for carotid endarterectomy.

On the day of surgery, metformin was omitted and hourly glucose measurements had started at 06:00. Premedication consisted of temazepam and his routine nifedipine orally at 07:00. An insulin infusion according to a sliding scale was also started in conjunction with a separate infusion of 0.1% normal saline in 4% dextrose at 100 ml/h. He arrived in the anaesthetic room at 09:00 where pulse oximetry and ECG monitoring with ST segment analysis were established. Under local anaesthesia a large-bore intravenous line and left radial arterial line were then inserted. Blood pressure was measured at 170/90 mmHg and heart rate was 85/min.

The patient was pre-oxygenated for 3 minutes and an infusion of esmolol was commenced. Anaesthesia was then induced with fentanyl and thiopentone. Vecuronium was administered to facilitate endotracheal intubation and anaesthesia was maintained with isoflurane in an air – oxygen mixture (FiO_2 0.4) with IPPV. After intubation the esmolol was discontinued and ventilation adjusted to give end tidal CO_2 readings of 4.5 kPa. A peripheral nerve stimulator was attached, nasopharyngeal temperature probe inserted, and a vecuronium infusion commenced to maintain neuromuscular blockade. The patient was then transferred to theatre.

Local anaesthetic was injected to the incision area by the surgeons, and heparin 5000 i.u. was given intravenously prior to vessel occlusion. Stump pressure was not measured by the surgeon as the practice in this unit was to insert a shunt in all patients (Fig. 33.1). Surgery was uneventful with all changes in blood pressure and heart rate being transient, not requiring any treatment with vaso-active agents. During the 2 hour procedure, blood sugar remained between 7–9 mmol/l.

On completion of surgery, anaesthesia was discontinued and neuromuscular blockade reversed with neostigmine and glycopyrrolate. Once spontaneous respiration was established, the patient was extubated and moved to the recovery room. On arrival in the recovery room he was drowsy but oriented and moving all four limbs to command. Invasive monitoring of blood pressure was continued and 6 l/min of oxygen administered through a Hudson mask. Two hours later, after return to the high dependency unit, blood pressure rose from an initial postoperative value of 145/85 mmHg to 190/95 mmHg. Sublingual nifedipine was given but there was only a small response, therefore an esmolol infusion was restarted. This was adjusted to maintain a blood pressure between 120 and 160 mmHg and was required for some 4 hours. Insulin on a sliding scale was continued overnight. The following morning he restarted normal oral intake and his usual medications were given. The

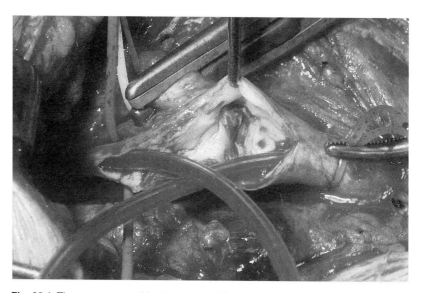

Fig. 33.1 The common carotid artery clamped (and opened) with the shunt in place

invasive monitoring was removed and the insulin infusion stopped. The remainder of his hospital stay was uncomplicated.

DISCUSSION POINTS

Both insulin-dependant and non-insulin-dependant diabetics are more likely to require surgery than their non-diabetic counterparts.

- *Question 1: What are the complications of diabetes that result in this?*

- *Question 2: Discuss the effects of anaesthesia and surgery on diabetes mellitus.*

There are several methods described to manage both insulin and non-insulin-dependant diabetes during the peri-operative period. One commonly used system was Alberti's Glucose – Insulin – Potassium regime, where all components were mixed into one infusion bag. Since then it has become common to give the insulin by a separate infusion, allowing different rates in response to blood sugar measurements. Even more recently a technique in which bolus doses of insulin are given in response to blood sugar measurements has been advocated by some centres.

- *Question 3: Discuss the advantages and disadvantages of these techniques.*

Carotid artery disease does not occur in isolation but almost invariably in association with other manifestations of vascular disease. Seventy percent of patients presenting for carotid surgery will have co-existing hypertension, the major risk factor for stroke. Myocardial ischaemia is also extremely common. Acute myocardial infarction is the most frequent cause of peri-operative mortality and morbidity in these patients.

- **Question 4:** *Discuss the pre-operative assessment of patients presenting for carotid artery surgery.*

The role of carotid endarterectomy in carotid artery disease is under continuing review. Occlusion of the vessel is necessary to allow surgical access during the procedure. In this case stump pressure was not measured as the practice of the surgeon was to insert a shunt in all patients with the aim of improving blood supply to the brain during the occlusion time. The assessment of neurological function and thus the ability to predict adequacy of cerebral perfusion – is an area of ongoing research. Various methods have been described.

- **Question 5:** *Can you discuss these methods, explain what stump pressure represents, and describe other methods which might be used to protect the brain from ischaemia during this procedure?*

This patient returned to the high-dependency unit, and postoperative care included invasive blood pressure monitoring.

- **Question 6:** *Discuss the major postoperative complications of this procedure and how they can be minimised.*

Local haemorrhage and haematoma formation at the operative site have also been reported.

● **Question 7:** *How would you recognise and deal with this complication?*

This case was carried out under general anaesthesia; however, carotid endarterectomy is routinely performed under local anaesthesia in some centres.

● **Question 8:** *Describe how you would do this and discuss the advantages and disadvantages of both regional and general techniques.*

FURTHER READING

Milaskiewicz R M, Hall G M. Diabetes and anaesthesia: the last decade. (editorial). Br J Anaes 1992; 68: 198–206

Hirsch I B, McGill J B, Cryer P E, White P F. Peri-operative management of surgical patients with diabetes mellitus. Anesthesiology 1991; 74: 346–359

Hall G M. Insulin administration in diabetic patients – the return of the bolus? Br J Anaes 1994; 72: 1–2

Garrioch M, Fitch W. Anaesthesia for carotid surgery. Br J Anaes 1993; 71: 569–579

European Carotid Surgery Trialists Collaborative Group IV European Carotid Artery Surgery Trial: Interim results for symptomatic patients with severe (70–99%) or with mild (0–29%) carotid stenosis. Lancet 1992; 337: 1235–1243

Bonnet F, Derosier J P, Pluskwa F, Abhay K, Gaillard A. Cervical epidural anaesthesia for carotid artery surgery. Can J Anaes 1990; 37: 353–358

Corson J D, Chang B B, Shah D M, Leather R P, DeLeo B M, Karmody A M. The influence of anaesthetic choice on carotid endarterectomy outcome. Arch Surg 1987; 122: 807–812

O'Sullivan J C, Wells D G, Wells G R. Difficult airway management with neck swelling after carotid endarterectomy. Anaesth Intensive Care 1986; 14: 460–464

34 Goitre and stridor

A 93-year-old woman presented with stridor. She had been previously well and currently took no medication. Apart from the obvious respiratory difficulty, physical examination was unremarkable. A chest X-ray revealed a severe narrowing of her trachea about 3 cm long, lying 3 cm above the carina (Fig. 34.2). Further investigation showed the stricture to be caused by a benign retrosternal goitre. Both clinically and biochemically she was euthyroid. Arterial blood gas analysis was normal apart from a PaO_2 of 9.2 kPa breathing air. In view of her age it was decided that the stricture should be dilated by introducing a stent into the trachea. This was to be introduced over a guide wire, using X-ray control, through an 8 mm endotracheal tube. Whilst awaiting this procedure she was given a helium – oxygen mixture to breathe via a face mask, with considerable relief of her symptoms. Breathing this mixture (FiO_2 0.3), the PaO_2 rose to 14.2 kPa. She was pre-medicated with glycopyrrolate intramuscularly one hour prior to the procedure.

A standard anaesthetic machine was adapted so as to allow the addition of a helium – oxygen mixture to the outflow from the vaporiser. A gas analyser was used to monitor halothane and oxygen levels of this mixture. A rigid bronchoscope and high-pressure oxygen source with standard connection were held in reserve.

After establishing basic monitoring, anaesthesia was induced using the halothane in the helium – oxygen mixture. Once it was confirmed the lungs could be ventilated via the face mask, small doses of alfentanil were administered whilst maintaining spontaneous ventilation. When anaesthesia was deep enough, a cuffed orotracheal tube was passed easily beyond the stricture and ventilation of both lungs confirmed. End tidal CO_2 monitoring was established. Spontaneous ventilation was assisted via the reservoir bag of a Magill type two coaxial system. Under X-ray control a guide wire was passed through the endotracheal tube and was seen to enter the right main bronchus. The patient was then given a halothane-in-oxygen mixture to breathe for 3 minutes. The endotracheal tube was withdrawn until the tip was above the stricture, the stent was then introduced and the guide wire withdrawn (Fig. 34.1 and 34.2). Introduction of the stent took 20 seconds, and at no time was the anaesthetist unable to ventilate both lungs. On recovery of gag reflex, the endotracheal tube was removed. Recovery was uneventful with complete resolution of symptoms.

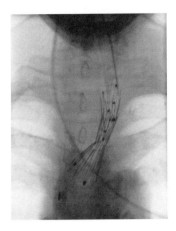 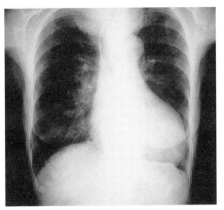

Fig. 34.1   **Fig. 34.2**

Fig. 34.1 & Fig. 34.2 X-rays showing examples of tracheal and bronchial stents

DISCUSSION POINTS

Airway obstruction due to goitre is usually thought to be rare. Radiographic evidence of tracheal compression is not uncommonly seen in such cases; however, the best method of establishing upper airway obstruction is the flow volume loop. This patient presented with stridor.

● *Question 1: What degree of loss of cross-sectional area would you expect before this symptom became apparent?*

● *Question 2: What other complications might result from retrosternal goitre?*

Instrumentation of the trachea in the presence of a stenosis will always carry a risk of obstruction. Major trans-sternal surgery will always carry a risk, particularly in this age group.

- *Question 3:* In view of these two statements, and given that the swelling was benign in this instance, discuss the treatment choice in this patient.

Awake intubation under local anaesthesia is said to be advantageous since the patient maintains the patency of the airway.

- *Question 4:* Do you think it would have been advisable to carry out this procedure under local anaesthesia?

- *Question 5:* Management of this patient involved breathing a helium – oxygen gas mixture. Why might this be thought to be beneficial in this case?

This patient presented with an anatomic complication of her thyroid disease. She was, however, euthyroid.

- *Question 6:* Discuss the management of the patient presenting with thyrotoxic crisis.

FURTHER READING

The thyroid cork. (editorial). Lancet 1990; 335: 1374–1375

Miller M R, Pincock A C, Oates G D, Wilkinson R, Skene-Smith H. Upper airway obstruction due to goitre: detection, prevalence and results of surgical management. Quarterly J Med 1990; 74: 177–188

Rudow M, Hill A B, Thompson N W et al. Helium – oxygen mixtures in airway obstruction due to thyroid carcinoma. Can Anaes Soc J 1986; 33: 498–501

Metabolic and anatomic thyroid emergencies: a review. Crit Care Med 1992; 20: 276–291

35 Airway laser surgery

A 75-year-old man presented to the local ENT department with hoarseness. Direct laryngoscopy and biopsy were performed under general anaesthesia and revealed a small laryngeal carcinoma. The surgeon planned to treat this with laser ablation.

The patient had a life-long history of cigarette smoking and on specific questioning admitted to exertional dyspnoea and angina. Examination revealed a cachectic patient, but there were no clinical signs of airway obstruction. Investigations included haematology, biochemistry, ECG and chest X-ray and confirmed a mild degree of anaemia, hypoproteinaemia and ischaemic heart disease but were otherwise unremarkable.

No premedication was given and after pre-oxygenation and the administration of glycopyrrolate, anaesthesia was induced with alfentanil and thiopentone. Muscle relaxation was achieved with vecuronium and the trachea was intubated with a flexible metallic nasotracheal tube with an internal diameter of 5.0 mm. The tube had two cuffs and these were both inflated with saline. Anaesthesia was maintained with isoflurane in nitrous oxide and oxygen. The laser was used in conjunction with a binocular microscope and suspension laryngoscope, and the procedure was carried out uneventfully.

DISCUSSION POINTS

The major hazard of airway laser surgery is that of airway fire. This is due to the locally high temperatures generated by the laser beam, the presence of combustible materials and the high oxygen concentrations found in the airway during anaesthesia. Combustion is not supported by volatile agents such as halothane, enflurane or isoflurane, but nitrous oxide supports combustion better than 100% oxygen.

- *Question 1: Why is a metallic endotracheal tube used, and why are the cuffs inflated with saline rather than air?*

● **Question 2:** *If a plastic tube has to be used, what precautions should be taken?*

● **Question 3:** *If the endotracheal tube is to be lubricated, what should or should not be used?*

An alternative technique would be to employ jet ventilation. This allows the surgeon a totally unobstructed field and avoids some of the problems associated with endotracheal tubes.

● **Question 4:** *What hazards does jet ventilation incur?*

● **Question 5:** *How would you maintain anaesthesia during jet ventilation?*

FURTHER READING

Conacher I D, Paes M C, Morritt G N. Anaesthesia for CO_2 laser surgery on the trachea. Br J Anaes 1985; 57: 448–450
Scammen F L, McCabe B F. Evaluation of supraglottic jet ventilation for laser surgery of the larynx. Anesthesiology 1984; 61: A447

Chilcoat R T, Byles P H, Kellam R M. The hazard of nitrous oxide during laser endoscopic surgery. Anesthesiology 1983; 59: 258

Keen R I, Kojak P K, Ramsden R T. Anaesthesia for microsurgery of the larynx. Ann RCSE 1982, 64, 111–113

Linscombe R M. Anaesthesia for microsurgery of the larynx. Ann RCSE 1982; 64: 430

Norton M L, Strong M S, Snow J C, Kripje B J. Endotracheal intubation and Venturi (jet) ventilation for laser microsurgery of the larynx. Ann Otolaryngol 1976; 85: 656–663

Ruder C B, Raphael N L, Abrahamson A L, Oliverio R M. Anaesthesia for carbon dioxide laser microsurgery of the larynx. Otolaryngology – Head and Neck Surgery 1981, 89, 732–737

Oliverio R M, Ruder C B, Abrahamson A L. Jet ventilation for laryngeal microsurgery. Br J Anaes 1981; 53: 1010

Vourch G, Tannieres M L, Freche G. Anaesthesia for microsurgery of the larynx using a carbon dioxide laser. Anaesthesia 1979; 34: 53–57

36 Anaphylaxis

A 32-year-old woman was admitted as a day case for the purpose of undergoing elective laparoscopy for investigation of chronic pelvic pain.

When seen by the anaesthetist she was fasted, and it was ascertained that she had arranged an escort and transport home. There was no significant past medical history, she had never had an anaesthetic before, was on no medications and had no known allergies. She was extremely anxious about the procedure and anaesthesia, but seemed somewhat reassured after talking with the anaesthetist and nursing staff. In the anaesthetic room basic monitoring was established; the ECG showed sinus rhythm with a heart rate of 102/min and the oxygen saturation was 98% breathing air. After two unsuccessful attempts at inserting venous cannulae, the anaesthetist inserted a butterfly needle into the dorsum of the hand. Her heart rate had risen to 120/min by this time and she had become tearful. Prior to induction she was again reassured.

Induction of anaesthesia proceeded with thiopentone, gallamine and suxamethonium. Immediately thereafter a widespread flare and wheal reaction involving the chest, neck and face developed. Tracheal intubation was rapidly performed, and despite mechanical ventilation with 100% oxygen, she became deeply cyanosed. Airway inflation pressure was noted to be high and the ECG monitor displayed ventricular tachycardia.

DISCUSSION POINTS

Both anaphylactic and anaphylactoid reactions can occur under general anaesthesia.

- *Question 1:* *What is the difference between these types of reactions and how are they mediated?*

● *Question 2:* *Can they be distinguished clinically?*

Most histamine in the body is present in the mast cells, although basophils, neurones and endothelial cells can also contain this substance. The half-life of histamine is less than one minute and so within a few minutes the resulting reaction to common drugs used during anaesthesia, such as opiates and atracurium, may be over. Histamine has effects on the skin, the cardiovascular and pulmonary systems.

● *Question 3:* *What are these effects and how are they mediated?*

● *Question 4:* *Can these effects be attenuated?*

● *Question 5:* *How would you proceed with resuscitation of this patient? Was induction of anaesthesia carried out in an acceptable manner?*

● *Question 6:* *What kind of follow-up to this reaction is necessary?*

FURTHER READING

Anaphylactoid reactions associated with anaesthesia. Report of a Working Party Association of Anaesthetists September 1990

Moudgil G C. Anaesthesia and allergic drug reactions. Can Anaes Soc J 1986; 33: 399–415

Moneret-Vautrin D A, Laxenaire M C. The risk of allergy related to general anaesthesia (review). Clin and Exp Allergy 1993; 23: 629–633

37 Pre-term labour

A previously healthy 20-year-old primigravida at 30 weeks gestation was admitted to the maternity unit in labour. Her membranes had ruptured spontaneously at home. Ritodrine hydrochloride was administered by intravenous infusion to inhibit uterine activity and intramuscular betamethasone commenced to accelerate foetal lung maturation.

As the woman was pyrexial (37.3°C) a high vaginal swab was taken, but antibiotic therapy withheld until the laboratory reported growth of a gram negative bacilli 13 hours later. Metronidazole and cefotaxime were prescribed. Meanwhile the ritodrine infusion had been gradually increased in an attempt to abolish the uterine contractions, but this had not been successful. The patient now began to complain of palpitations. Her pulse rate was recorded at 112/min. She was reassured this was a common side-effect of the drug. However, when she complained of feeling breathless the infusion rate was reduced but not stopped. Several hours later she was not only markedly breathless but now also cyanosed. When a pulse oximeter was attached to the patient, oxygen saturation was measured as 80%. The ritodrine was discontinued and high flow oxygen administered by face mask. At this point she was examined vaginally and her cervix found to be fully dilated. Shortly thereafter she was delivered of a live infant with minimal blood loss. The infant was attended by a paediatrician and quickly transferred to the special care nursery. Oxytocin was given intravenously before the placenta was expelled.

Following delivery she became more dyspnoeic and distressed. Auscultation of her chest revealed widespread bilateral crepitations. A working diagnosis of left ventricular failure caused by excessive sympathetic stimulation was made. Frusemide was administered intravenously, followed by propranolol and morphine. Despite a diuresis of 2 L over the ensuing 2 hours, the patient remained in marked respiratory distress. Her core temperature was now 39.7°C and peripheral white cell count reported as $48.0 \times 10^9/l$. A chest X-ray was consistent with extensive bilateral pulmonary oedema and arterial blood gases confirmed severe hypoxaemia, with acidosis and mild hypercapnia (PaO_2 3.4 kPa, pH 7.14, and $PaCO_2$ 5.6 kPa). Her pulse rate remained rapid at 140/min with systolic blood pressure varying between 70–80 mmHg. At this point she was intubated, ventilated with 100% oxygen and an infusion of dopamine commenced to produce a pressure of 90 mmHg systolic. Transfer was arranged to the intensive care unit.

DISCUSSION POINTS

This woman developed severe pulmonary oedema while receiving a β adrenergic agonist in an attempt to inhibit uterine activity. The incidence of pulmonary oedema with the use of these drugs has been reported as high as 5% in one study. While the pulmonary oedema is usually readily reversible, there has been a fatal outcome in at least nine cases.

• *Question 1:* *Discuss the presentation and management of pulmonary oedema in such a case in the obstetric unit.*

There are several factors in this woman's case which increase her risk of pulmonary oedema with the use of a β adrenergic agonist.

• *Question 2:* *Can you identify these?*

• *Question 3:* *What other factors may be associated with an increased risk?*

The infant in this case is also in a high-risk category. There are both the risks of prematurity and sepsis.

- **Question 4:** *Describe the equipment necessary in the delivery room for resuscitation of the neonate, and the routine assessment and management of the neonate in the immediate post-delivery period.*

FURTHER READING

Chestnut D H, Dailey P A. Anesthesia for preterm labour and delivery. In: Schnider S M, Levinson C, eds. Anesthesia for obstetrics. 3rd ed. Baltimore: Williams and Wilkins, 1993: 341–350

Graf R A, Perez Woods R. Trends in preterm labor. J Perinatol 1992; 19: 367–384

Grand Rounds – Hammersmith Hospital. β Adrenergic agonists and pulmonary oedema in preterm labour. BMJ 1994; 308: 260–262

Harless F E. The use of tocolytics in patients with preterm premature rupture of the membranes. Clin Obstet Gynecol 1991; 34: 751–758

Bendetti T J. Complications of betamimetic therapy. Clin Perinatol 1986; 13: 843–852

Elliott R D. Neonatal resuscitation: The NRP guidelines. Can J Anaes 1994; 41: 742–753

38 Myotonic dystrophy in pregnancy

A 28-year-old pregnant woman presented at 34 weeks gestation in her second pregnancy. Myotonic dystrophy had been diagnosed two years previously and her condition had deteriorated significantly during this pregnancy. She had been delivered of her first child by emergency caesarean section under epidural anaesthesia following the development of foetal distress in labour. The post-partum period had been complicated by depression and a pulmonary embolism at 8 weeks post-delivery. She had suffered a deep-vein thrombosis 6 years previously and was on long-term warfarin therapy. In addition, she suffered from asthma and used salbutamol and beclomethasone inhalers.

Since the diagnosis of myotonic dystrophy was made she had twice had dental extractions under general anaesthesia. On each occasion anaesthesia was induced with propofol and endotracheal intubation accomplished without the use of a muscle relaxant. Anaesthesia was maintained with a mixture of isoflurane in nitrous oxide and oxygen with spontaneous respiration.

Elective caesarean section was planned for 37 weeks. The obstetrician sought anaesthetic advice in order to work out a plan of action to cover the elective procedure and any emergency situations which might arise.

On meeting the patient, the anaesthetist noted she was sitting in a wheelchair. She displayed the characteristic myotonic facies with wasting of the facial muscles and frontal balding. Physical examination revealed a myotonic grip in the left hand and decreased power in all four limbs with reduced reflexes. Examination of the chest and cardiovascular system was unremarkable.

Further clinical investigations were obtained. These consisted of an electrocardiograph, a chest X-ray, echocardiography, arterial blood gas analysis and pulmonary function tests. The results of these investigations were all within normal limits apart from the pulmonary function tests. These showed an obstructive ventilatory defect with reduction in functional residual capacity, vital capacity and total lung capacity.

The problems faced were two-fold: this was a patient on long-term anti-coagulation facing major surgery on a planned date but who might require urgent caesarean section if she went into pre-term labour. Secondly, the patient was asthmatic and suffered from a multi-system disorder which would significantly complicate the course of an anaesthetic.

After discussion with the obstetrician, the following management was agreed. Warfarin would be discontinued at 36 weeks gestation and heparin anticoagulation commenced. Prothrombin time (PT) and subsequently activated partial thromboplastin time (APTT) would be monitored daily and dosages adjusted to maintain the desired degree of anticoagulation, that is, an APTT 1.5–2 times the midpoint of the normal range. Heparin therapy would be stopped 24 hours prior to surgery, and following a normal anticoagulation screen an epidural catheter would be inserted and used to provide anaesthesia for surgery and postoperative analgesia. She would be closely monitored postoperatively in a high dependency unit. Anticoagulation would be restarted immediately post-surgery, with heparin initially until the patient can take warfarin orally, and allowing for a 3-day overlap.

If labour started before the planned date of Caesarean Section or if emergency general anaesthesia was required, it was agreed that anaesthesia would be induced with propofol and the trachea would be intubated without the use of a muscle relaxant. Anaesthesia would be maintained with a continuous infusion of propofol and elective post-operative ventilation would be undertaken in the Intensive Care Unit.

Vitamin K and fresh-frozen plasma would be administered to reverse warfarin. Heparin would simply be discontinued and should bleeding be a problem, residual heparin reversed with protamine.

DISCUSSION POINTS

• **Question 1:** *Myotonic dystrophy is a multi-system disorder, extra muscular involvement is inevitable. Which systems are involved, and how should your pre-operative investigations reflect this?*

• **Question 2:** *Ventilatory involvement in myotonic dystrophy is multi-factorial. What factors are involved, and how will this affect anaesthetic management?*

- **Question 3:** *There is an association with myotonic dystrophy and malignant hyperthermia. How will this alter the conduct of anaesthesia?*

- **Question 4:** *Myotonic dystrophy is associated with uterine hypotonia and increased risk of post-partum haemorrhage. How would you prepare for this?*

- **Question 5:** *Discuss the relative risks to mother and foetus of warfarin and heparin therapy.*

- **Question 6:** *If following the cessation of heparin therapy the APTT remains abnormal, is spinal anaesthesia an option?*

FURTHER READING

Blumgart C H, Hughes D G, Redfern N. Obstetric anaesthesia in dystrophia myotonica. Anaesthesia 1990; 45: 26–29

Russell S H, Hirsch N P. Anaesthesia and myotonia. Br J Anaes 1994; 72: 210–216

Howell P R, Douglas J M. Lupus anticoagulant, paramyotonia congenita and pregnancy. Can J Anaes 1992; 39: 992–996

Ogawa K, Iranami Y, Yoshiyama T, Maeda H, Hatano Y. Severe respiratory depression after epidural morphine in a patient with myotonic dystrophy. Can J Anaes 1993; 40: 968–70

Aldridge L M. Anaesthetic problems in myotonic dystrophy: a case report and review of the Aberdeen experience compromising 48 general anaesthetics in a further 16 patients. Br J Anaes 1985; 57: 1119–1130

Mudge B J, Taylor P B, Vanderspek A F L. Perioperative hazards in myotonic dystrophy. Anaesthesia 1980; 35: 492–495

Paterson R A, Tousignant M, Skene D S. Caesarean section for twins in a patient with myotonic dystrophy. Can Anaes Soc J 1985; 32: 418–421

Wille-Jorgensen P, Jorgensen L N, Rasmussen L S. Lumbar regional anaesthesia and prophylactic anticoagulant therapy. Anaesthesia 1991; 46: 623–627

Wildsmith J A W, McClure J H. Anticoagulant drugs and central nerve blockade. Anaesthesia 1991; 46: 613–614

Hughes S M. Anaesthesia for the pregnant patient with neuromuscular disorders. In: Shnider S M, Levinson G, eds. Anaesthesia for obstetrics. 3rd ed. Baltimore: Williams and Wilkins, 1993: 581–595

Maternal and neonatal haemostasis working party of the haemostasis and thrombosis task force. Guidelines on the prevention, investigation and management of thrombosis associated with pregnancy. J Clinical Path 1993; 46: 489–496

39

Multiple sclerosis in pregnancy

A 29-year-old primagravida with a clinical diagnosis of multiple sclerosis and variable sensory loss of sensation to pinprick and paraesthesia in the right upper and left lower limb wished to be awake during her emergency caesarean section for failure to progress.

On closer questioning, it was ascertained that her problems began 2 years previously with visual disturbances which had now settled, but the symptoms of variable weakness in her right arm and left leg had been present for over a year and became slightly worse during pregnancy. She had been diagnosed by a neurologist one year after the onset of symptoms and 3 months before becoming pregnant.

She wished to know if there were any risks associated with an 'epidural' because she had been told that 'a general anaesthetic would make the multiple sclerosis worse'. She was obese and had never had an anaesthetic or operation before. She had good mouth opening. She had been in labour for 20 hours and was tired but insistent on staying awake if possible. After a full explanation of the various anaesthetic options was given to her, she and the anaesthetist made a joint decision to proceed to caesarean section under spinal anaesthetic.

A full aseptic technique was adhered to, and bupivacaine 0.5% hyperbaric mixed with fentanyl was introduced to the subarachnoid space at the L3/4 level after a single puncture with a 25 G Whitacre pencil-point needle. Surgical anaesthesia was quickly established and the operation proceeded uneventfully. At review 8 hours later, she felt the weakness in her foot was slightly worse and that in her hand was slightly better. At 24 hours the hand remained slightly better, but the foot was no worse or better than pre-operatively.

DISCUSSION POINTS

The course of a de-myelinating disease during pregnancy is variable, but there is some evidence that the relapse rate is higher during pregnancy. The need for anaesthetic and obstetric intervention for this patient makes the situation even less clear. The options for this particular patient are: general anaesthesia; epidural anaesthesia; and spinal anaesthesia.

- *Question 1:* *What would you tell this patient about the relative benefits and risks of these techniques?*

- *Question 2:* *It is possible to carry out a caesarean section using infiltration of local anaesthetic into the abdominal wall. Do you think that this is a reasonable proposition?*

- *Question 3:* *Do you think that it is wise to add fentanyl to the solution of bupivacaine? Would you prefer to administer another opioid instead?*

- *Question 4:* *What advantages accrue and what are the potential adverse effects?*

FURTHER READING

Korn-Lubetski I, Kahana E, Cooper G, Abramsky O. Activity of multiple sclerosis during pregnancy and the puerperium. Ann Neurology 1984; 16: 299–231
Bamford C, Sibley W, Laguna J. Anaesthesia in multiple sclerosis. Can J Neurolog Sciences 1978; 5: 41–44

Bader A M, Hunt C O, Datta S, Naulty S, Ostheimer G W. Anesthesia for the obstetric patient with multiple sclerosis. J Clinical Anes 1988; 1: 21–24

Alderson J D. Intrathecal diamorphine and multiple sclerosis (letter). Anaesthesia 1990; 45: 1084–1085

40

A 27-year-old primigravida at 34 weeks gestation in a previously uneventful pregnancy developed increasing breathlessness on exertion over the course of 2 days. She consulted her general practitioner when the dyspnoea became so severe that she was no longer able to climb the stairs at home without stopping for a rest. On examination she was found to have a respiratory rate of 30 breaths/min at rest, but auscultation revealed no abnormality. She had mild peripheral oedema and her blood pressure was 130/90 mmHg. She was unable to produce a specimen of urine and remarked that she could not remember voiding urine since the previous day. The GP was sufficiently worried to arrange urgent admission to the maternity hospital where these clinical findings were confirmed, and it was noted she had a dry unproductive cough. A chest X-ray showed signs of interstitial pulmonary oedema and an enlarged heart with left ventricular prominence. Oxygen saturation on air was 92% but was raised to 99% when she was given 4 l of oxygen to breathe by face mask. A urinary catheter was passed and drained 50 ml of urine which showed large amounts of protein on testing. A diagnosis of pre-eclampsia was made. An intravenous line was inserted and 1 L of 0.9% saline infused over 30 minutes.

It was decided to deliver her by caesarean section. In theatre after establishing routine monitoring, the patient was tilted slightly head down, while maintaining the left lateral tilt, and the anaesthetist inserted a central venous pressure line by the right subclavian route. This read 9 cm H_2O. Before any further action was taken, she developed severe respiratory distress, oxygen saturation fell to 80% and she began to cough up frothy pink sputum. She was intubated following a rapid-sequence intravenous induction of anaesthesia. Despite delivery of 100% oxygen, the pulse oximeter failed to read above 90%. Her blood pressure read 70 mmHg and the foetal heart rate had fallen acutely to 80/min. The obstetrician wished to perform the caesarean section immediately and the anaesthetist agreed.

During the procedure the anaesthetist was able to exchange the central venous line for a pulmonary artery catheter. The mean pulmonary artery pressure was recorded as 30 mmHg and the pulmonary artery occlusion pressure 22 mmHg. A live infant was delivered and after initial resuscitation in theatre was transferred to the special care nursery.

Following the caesarean section the patient was kept intubated and ventilated and transferred to the intensive care unit. Intravenous infusions

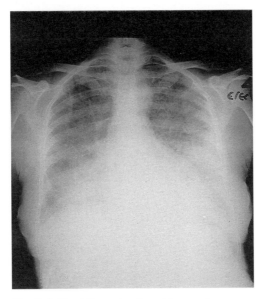

Fig. 40.1 Chest X-ray showing widespread pulmonary oedema

of dopamine and adrenaline were required to maintain a blood pressure of 100 mmHg but despite this she remained oliguric. The chest X-ray now showed bilateral pulmonary oedema (Fig. 40.1), and blood gases (FiO$_2$ 1.0) revealed a PO$_2$ of 9.6 kPa and a metabolic acidosis. Echocardiography displayed a poorly contracting dilated left ventricle (ejection fraction 35%) with some mitral regurgitation. Management was supportive with continued inotrope infusion and strict fluid restriction.

Forty eight hours later, oxygenation had improved markedly, the inotropic support had been discontinued and she began to produce large volumes of urine. Over the subsequent 24 hours she was weaned from the ventilator and extubated. Repeat echocardiography reflected the improved myocardial function, and there was no longer any mitral regurgitation. She continued to progress rapidly to a complete recovery.

DISCUSSION POINTS

This patient presented acutely with pre-eclampsia. This pathology was first described over 100 years ago and yet the precise pathophysiology remains unclear.

- **Question 1:** *How do you interpret this patient's history in terms of the current understanding of the pathophysiology of pre-eclampsia?*

Pulmonary oedema is a serious development in a patient with pre-eclampsia.

- **Question 2:** *What other ominous signs and symptoms should be watched for?*

- **Question 3:** *What is the HELLP syndrome?*

- **Question 4:** *This patient had significantly different central venous pressure and pulmonary artery occlusion pressure measurements. Is this a recognised feature of severe pre-eclampsia?*

- **Question 5:** *What are the reasons for oliguria in the pre-eclamptic patient?*

- **Question 6:** *Do you think the early management in this case contributed to the subsequent course of events?*

- **Question 7:** *How can you be sure that a fluid challenge is safe or even appropriate in such a presentation?*

- **Question 8:** *Describe the cardiovascular changes found in the pregnant woman.*

- **Question 9:** *What would you expect the central venous pressure to read in a normal pregnancy?*

- **Question 10:** *What is the most frequent cause of maternal mortality in the pre-eclamptic woman?*

FURTHER READING

Nolan T E, Wakefield M L, Devoe L D. Invasive hemodynamic monitoring in obstetrics. Chest 1992; 101: 1428–1433

Cunningham F G, Lindheimer M D. Hypertension in pregnancy. N Eng J Med 1992; 326: 927–932

Harris A P. General anaesthesia and toxemia of pregnancy. Anes Analg 1992; 75: 150–152

Cotton D B, Gonik B, Dorman K, Harrist R. Cardiovascular complication in severe pregnancy-induced hypertension: relationship of central venous pressure to pulmonary capillary wedge pressure. Am J Obstet Gynecol 1985; 151: 762–764

Clark S L, Greenspoon J S, Aldahl D, Phelan J P. Severe pre-eclampsia with persistent oliguria: management of hemodynamic subsets. Am J Obstet Gynecol 1986; 154: 490–494

Bendetti M D, Kates R, Williams V. Hemodynamic observations in severe pre-eclampsia complicated by pulmonary edema. Am J Obstet Gynecol 1985; 152: 330–334

Pearson J F. Fluid balance in severe pre-eclampsia. Br J Hosp Med 1992; 48: 47–51

Phelan J P, Yuruth D A. Severe pre-eclampsia: peripartum hemodynamic considerations. Am J Obstet Gynecol 1982; 144: 17–22

41 Neuroblastoma

A four-year-old girl presented with a history of excessive sweating. Her past medical history included the usual febrile illnesses of childhood. Systematic enquiry revealed only that she appeared to have started to sweat excessively about 3 months earlier. Examination revealed bilateral proptosis, significant hypertension and the presence of a large central tumour in the abdomen.

A provisional diagnosis of neuroblastoma was supported by elevated urinary levels of hydroxymethoxymandelic acid and homovanillic acid. MRI scan of her abdomen revealed a large tumour apparently arising from the left adrenal medulla. MRI scan of her head revealed bilateral retro-orbital tumour. The combination of large tumour size and retro-orbital metastasis placed her in Stage IV of the disease as defined by the criteria of Evans, D'Angio and Randolph.

The general anaesthetic for the 40 minute MRI scan had been uneventful. Her blood pressure remained elevated but stable at 135/90 mmHg.

She was scheduled for laparotomy for excision of the primary tumour. Pre-operative investigations included serum electrolytes, full blood count and chest X-ray. Blood pressure remained elevated at 140–160/90 mmHg. In view of her hypertension a 12-lead ECG was recorded, which was normal. Apart from the excessive sweating, she remained asymptomatic.

Premedication consisted of trimeprazine orally and EMLA cream to the dorsum of one hand 2 hours pre-operatively. Anaesthesia was induced with thiopentone and fentanyl, and muscle relaxation provided with vecuronium. Following tracheal intubation, anaesthesia was maintained with isoflurane and nitrous oxide in oxygen. A radial arterial cannula was inserted for continuous blood pressure monitoring. Large-bore venous access was secured and a urinary catheter placed prior to transfer into theatre.

During the laparotomy, marked hypertension (up to 200/130 mmHg) was produced during tumour mobilisation. This was treated with incremental doses of labetalol, and the systolic blood pressure was maintained below 160 mmHg. Additional fentanyl was administered as a bolus intravenous dose. After a period of stability, systolic blood pressure again rose to 190 mmHg with an associated short period of ventricular bigeminy. Further treatment with labetalol successfully resolved both.

Following clamping of the venous drainage of the tumour, the troublesome hypertension subsided. Indeed, blood pressure dropped to 85 mmHg systolic and required colloid replacement of the intra-operative blood loss to restore normal levels. The procedure was completed uneventfully, anaesthesia was discontinued and once full neuromuscular function and spontaneous respiration had returned, she was extubated. She was transferred to the recovery room where an infusion of morphine was commenced to control postoperative pain. Oxygen was delivered by face mask and the arterial cannula was removed.

The recovery room nurses alerted the anaesthetist to two problems: the child's axillary temperature was 35.4°C and no urine was present in the collecting device which had not been emptied since the time of catheter insertion.

The child was covered with a space blanket and a rapid infusion of PPS was administered through an infusion warmer. Her temperature rose steadily and she began to produce urine over the next hour. One hour later she was transferred to the ward. Overnight she required further fluid replacement with blood and PPS to maintain adequate urine production. As the oximeter displayed a fall in S_pO_2 to 93% on air, oxygen by face mask was continued for 48 hours.

On the first postoperative day, cardiovascular variables were stable and urine production was good. Pain control was satisfactory with the morphine infusion, but she was too drowsy to co-operate well with the physiotherapist on that day. By the second postoperative day her drowsiness had diminished enough to allow full co-operation. She made a slow but steady recovery.

DISCUSSION POINTS

This child presented with hypertension, for which a cause was found.

● *Question 1:* *In view of her subsequent course, what pre-operative treatment might have been indicated, and what other treatment might have reduced the risk of intra-operative hypertension?*

Her intra-operative hypertension was treated with labetalol. This drug has both alpha-blocking and beta-blocking activity.

- *Question 2:* Does the action of this drug pose any potential hazard when used for control of hypertension in these circumstances?

- *Question 3:* Which alternative agents might be used for rapid control of hypertension?

A long laparotomy in a small child can easily result in significant heat loss.

- *Question 4:* What are the modes of this heat loss and what measures could you take to counteract this?

Management of postoperative pain in this child was with an intravenous morphine infusion.

- *Question 5:* Can you discuss the advantages and disadvantages of this method and suggest other methods of pain control in this age of child?

● **Question 6:** *What advantages and disadvantages might each have in this case?*

FURTHER READING

Creagh-Barry P, Sumner E. Neuroblastoma and anaesthesia. Paed Anaes 1992; 2: 147–152
Finkelstein J Z. Neuroblastoma: the challenge and frustration. Haematol/Oncol Clin N Am 1987; 1: 675–693
Evans A E, D'Angelo G J, Randolph J. A proposed staging for children with neuroblastoma. Cancer 1971; 27: 374–378

42 Acute burn

A three-year-old child was brought into the Accident and Emergency (A&E) Department having sustained 25% burns involving the chin, neck, chest and abdomen. One hour previously whilst playing with matches in her mother's bedroom her night-dress caught fire. Her screams alerted her mother, who smothered the flames with a quilt and dowsed the girl under the shower before calling for an ambulance.

The anaesthetic registrar on call was asked to assist in her initial resuscitation and early management. The A&E staff required assistance in assessing and managing the airway and breathing, circulation, fluid requirements and analgesia.

On arrival in the A&E department the anaesthetist noted that she was crying and opening her eyes to voice. She was cold, shivery and still partially dressed in the burnt clothing. Her lips were pink and the respiratory rate was 30/min. There was no stridor or other evidence of respiratory distress. Auscultation revealed good bilateral air entry with no added sounds. The burns to her chest were not circumferential. A pulse oximeter placed on a foot showed an oxygen saturation of 95%. A nurse was asked to hold an oxygen mask to her face in order to administer high-flow oxygen.

Her heart rate was 140/min, and her blood pressure measured on a thigh cuff was 100/65 mmHg. Peripheral pulses were all palpable; however, the extremities looked pale, felt cool, and capillary refill on her feet was five seconds. The anaesthetist decided the first priority was to obtain intravenous access. The A&E staff had attempted venous cannulation but, given the peripheral vasoconstriction and burn distribution were unsuccessful. The anaesthetist elected to insert an intra-osseous needle into the tibia (Figs 42.1, 42.2). This was accomplished under local anaesthesia. Bone marrow was aspirated and samples were sent to the laboratory for cross-matching of four units of blood and haemoglobin, haematocrit, blood sugar, urea and electrolytes.

The child's weight was estimated as 14 kg based on the formula $2 \times (age + 4) = weight (kg)$, and she was given an initial 20 ml/kg bolus of PPS via a syringe through the intra-osseous needle. To provide analgesia morphine was also administered by this route and a urinary catheter was inserted.

Throughout the assessment every effort was made to keep the child warm by removing damp clothing and, when not being examined, exposed areas were covered with sterile towels.

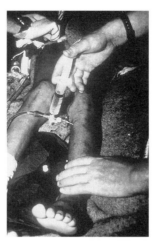

Fig. 42.1

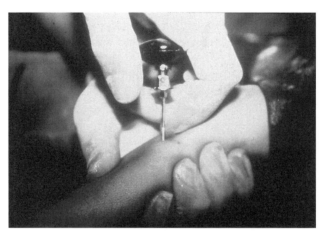

Fig. 42.2

Fig. 42.1 & Fig. 42.2 Photographs of intraosseous needle in use

At this point the plastic surgeon arrived. Now that the initial resuscitation and assessment had been accomplished, he felt she needed transfer to the intensive care unit. This would permit the insertion of a central venous and arterial line and a period of further assessment before she underwent debridement and grafting of burns.

The anaesthetic registrar requested the help of a senior colleague, and preparations were made for transfer to the intensive care unit.

DISCUSSION POINTS

The most common cause of death within the first hour following burn injuries is smoke inhalation. Administration of high concentrations of oxygen is important in the management of these patients, and it may be necessary to intubate the patient to do this, or to protect the airway. Although this child received high-flow oxygen through a face mask, a decision not to intubate this child in the A&E department was made.

- *Question 1:* *What factors should influence this decision, and which burns patients should be intubated at an early stage in their management?*

The intra-osseous route was used to obtain access as an initial emergency measure, although eschar can be perforated to provide intravenous access if necessary. The intra-osseous route was used in this case to sample, to administer fluid and to administer drugs.

- *Question 2:* *Can you discuss the equipment required for this procedure, the landmarks to be used, the types of patients it can be used in, and the advantages and disadvantages of this route as compared to standard intravenous access?*

- *Question 3:* *Are there any contra-indications to its use?*

An initial bolus of fluid was given to treat shock.

- *Question 4:* *How would you calculate subsequent fluid requirements and monitor the efficacy of fluid therapy?*

Some older children may be able to use Entonox. In this case morphine was used to provide analgesia.

● **Question 5:** *What other methods of pain relief might be suitable, and how would you provide continuing analgesia if presented with this case?*

Hypothermia is a significant problem in patients with severe burns.

● **Question 6:** *How can a burn patient be safely re-warmed, and what steps would you take in order to minimise further heat loss?*

This patient may make many trips to the operating theatre in the course of treatment for her burns.

● **Question 7:** *Briefly consider the physiological and psychological implications of this and the effect this will have on how you would anaesthetise this child.*

FURTHER READING

Muir M J, Herndon D N. The challenge of burns (review). Lancet 1994; 343: 216–220
Cote C J. Burn debridement. In: Stehling L, ed. Common problems in paediatric anaesthesia. St Louis: Mosby-Year Book, 1992: 207–218
Hain W R. The role of the anaesthetist in burns care. In: Judkins K C, ed. Burns and plastic surgery. London: Balliere Tindall, 1987; I: 565–573
Advanced paediatric life support: the practical approach. London: BMJ Publishing, 1993
Kruse J A, Vyskocil J J, Haupt M T. Intraosseous infusions. Crit Care Med 1994; 22: 728–729
Fiser D H. Intraosseous infusion. N Eng J Med 1990; 322: 1579–1581

43 MRI scan

A 5-year-old 20 kg boy with a diagnosis of idiopathic epilepsy presented for an MRI scan because of increasing frequency of fits over the preceding 3 months and the development of lethargy and tiredness. The child had a history of grand mal seizures starting from about the age of 1 year. The seizures were well controlled with phenytoin and sodium valproate. Initially the seizures were thought to be related to febrile illnesses, however, an EEG proved to be abnormal and a diagnosis of idiopathic epilepsy was made. A CT scan at that time was normal, as were all other screening investigations. General development was normal, and he had just started at his local primary school. He had no other medical problems.

General examination revealed a pleasant, co-operative boy. He was apyrexial and physical examination was normal; in particular, there were no neurological signs and no papilloedema. In addition to the MRI scan, other investigations included blood sugar, haemoglobin and full blood count, anti-convulsant levels, urea, electrolytes, creatinine and liver function tests, calcium and phosphate levels, blood culture, virology, chest X-ray, evoked potentials and EEG. The paediatrician asked the anaesthetist to take the necessary blood samples.

The MRI scan involved lying still for up to 30 minutes in an enclosed, noisy space, which few children below the age of 8 years will tolerate. There might also be the need for an intravenous injection of contrast medium. In view of the recent history of headache, and therefore the possibility of raised intracranial pressure, the anaesthetist felt that general anaesthesia was more appropriate than heavy sedation.

EMLA cream was applied topically to the dorsum of one hand 90 minutes before the scan. The patient was anaesthetised outside the scan room. Following the insertion of an intravenous cannula, anaesthesia was induced using thiopentone, and atracurium was given to facilitate endotracheal intubation. Following hyperventilation with 50% nitrous oxide and isoflurane 0.5% in oxygen, the trachea was intubated with a size 5.0 mm internal diameter RAE preformed endotracheal tube. Anaesthesia was maintained using the same mixture.

The patient was checked for any remaining metal objects in contact, a length of injection tubing was flushed through with saline and attached to his intravenous cannula, and he was then transported to the scan room (Fig. 1, Fig. 2). Mechanical ventilation was provided using an extended co-axial circuit and an MRI compatible Ventipac ventilator. Monitoring of ECG, non-invasive blood pressure, end-tidal carbon dioxide, oxygen

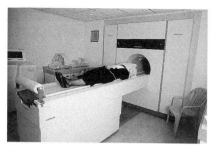 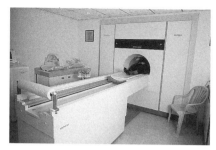

Fig. 43.1   **Fig. 43.2**

Fig. 43.1 & Fig. 43.2 Photographs of set up in MRI scan room with an unanaesthetised adult

saturation and skin temperature was carried out with MRI-compatible equipment and placed on appropriate sites to avoid image degradation due to the introduction of stray radiofrequency currents. Care was taken with the positioning of cables to avoid patient skin burns. The scan took 20 minutes; halfway through, contrast medium was injected – gadolinium pentolate. The patient was removed from the scanner and taken out to the anaesthetic area for reversal of anaesthesia and recovery.

The whole scan proceeded uneventfully and the child woke normally. The subsequent scan report stated that no abnormality had been detected.

DISCUSSION POINTS

The whole body magnet which forms the basis of the scanner is permanently 'on', therefore all ferromagnetic objects must be excluded from the field unless they are secured.

- *Question 1:* *What are the units of measurement of magnetic field strength?*

- *Question 2:* *Within what range do clinical scanners operate? Can you correlate this to the strength of the earth's magnetic field?*

The bore of the magnet is narrow, severely restricting patient access, and very little of the patient can be seen. Access to the patient may be further reduced by the use of head or surface coils. In addition, the operation of the gradient coils produces a loud thumping noise.

- *Question 3:* *In view of these constraints, is sedation rather than general anaesthesia a reasonable proposition?*

Monitoring equipment and leads can seriously degrade image quality by introducing stray radiofrequency currents, and conversely monitoring equipment will malfunction due to the changing magnetic field gradients.

- *Question 4:* *How can this be avoided?*

- *Question 5:* *What precautions would you take to avoid inducing skin burns from the monitoring cables?*

- *Question 6:* *Consider what manoeuvres might be necessary should the patient in the scanner urgently require cardiopulmonary resuscitation, e.g. sudden onset of ventricular fibrillation or an acute anaphylactic reaction to the contrast medium.*

FURTHER READING

Shellock F G, Kanal E. Patient monitoring during clinical MR imaging. Radiology 1992; 185: 623–629

Patteson S K, Chesney J T. Anaesthetic management for magnetic resonance imaging: problems and solutions. Anes and Analg 1992; 74: 121–128

Menon D K, Peden C J, Hall A S, Sargentoni J, Whitwam J G. Magnetic resonance for the anaesthetist. Part I: physical principles, applications, safety aspects. Anaesthesia 1992; 47: 240–255

Peden C J, Menon D K, Hall A S, Sargentoni J, Whitwam J G. Magnetic resonance for the anaesthetist. Part II: anaesthesia and monitoring in MR units. Anaesthesia 1992; 47: 508–517

Sury M R J, Johnstone G, Bingham R M. Anaesthesia for magnetic resonance imaging of children. Paed Anaes 1992; 2: 61–68

Taber K H, Thompson J, Coveler L A, Hayman L A. Invasive pressure monitoring of patients during magnetic resonance imaging. Can J Anaes 1993; 40: 1092–1095

Vangerven M, van Hemelrijck J, Wouters P, Vandermeesch E, van Aken H. Light anaesthesia with propofol for paediatric MRI. Anaesthesia 1992; 47: 706–707

Langton J A, Wilson I, Fell D. Use of the laryngeal mask airway during magnetic resonance imaging. Anaesthesia 1992; 47: 532

Crofts S, Campbell A. A source of artefact during general anaesthesia for magnetic resonance imaging. Anaesthesia 1993; 48: 643

Magnetic resonance imaging in epilepsy. (editorial.) Lancet 1992; 340: 343

Mosely I. Safety and magnetic resonance imaging. (editorial.) BMJ 1994, 308, 1181–2

44 Gastroschisis

A two-hour-old baby presented for repair of gastroschisis. The baby was born by spontaneous vaginal delivery, an intrauterine diagnosis of the condition having been made. The surgeon was anxious to proceed with surgery as soon as possible, as the blood supply to part of the bowel was thought to be compromised.

In preparation for the procedure the theatre temperature was set to increase to 28°C and a warming blanket placed on the operating table set to 38°C. The baby was brought to theatre in an incubator with the lower half of its body in a plastic body bag. The baby was breathing air spontaneously, there was no evidence of respiratory distress, and an oxygen saturation monitor on the hand displayed a reading of 97%. An oro-gastric tube deflated the stomach. Two intravenous infusions were running through a cannula on the dorsum of the left hand. One infusion was a maintenance volume of 0.18% saline in 10% dextrose, the other an infusion of 10 ml/kg of plasma protein solution (PPS). The baby's weight was 2.4 kg, temperature 36.8°C, blood sugar 3.5 mmol/l, and the haemoglobin, urea and electrolytes were within normal limits. One unit of packed cells was cross-matched and available.

As soon as preparations were complete and the theatre warmed, the baby was removed from the incubator to the operating table and monitoring equipment (consisting of ECG, non-invasive blood pressure and oxygen saturation monitor) were attached. Following pre-oxygenation, anaesthesia was induced with thiopentone and suxamethonium was administered to facilitate passage of a 3 mm uncuffed endotracheal tube. Following auscultation of the chest the endotracheal tube was secured 9 cm at the lips. End tidal CO_2 monitoring was instituted and a combined oesophageal stethoscope with temperature probe was inserted into the oesophagus. Mechanical ventilation was continued throughout with a mixture of warmed and humidified oxygen in air, with the addition of isoflurane. Atracurium and fentanyl were administered prior to the start of surgery. Every effort was made to minimise heat loss during induction. The head was wrapped, as were all four limbs. Warm fluid was used for skin cleaning. An additional intravenous cannula was inserted into the right hand.

Initially, surgery proceeded uneventfully. Multiple boluses of 2 ml/kg lactated Ringers solution and 4.5% PPS were administered to replace evaporative and third-space losses. The abdominal wall was stretched, and it proved possible to return the abdominal contents entirely. However, at the time of abdominal closure there was a marked increase in intra-abdominal pressure. This was accompanied by a reduction in respiratory compliance and cardiac output, an increase in inflation pressure, fall in oxygen saturation and reduction in blood pressure. After a few minutes the respiratory and cardiac parameters stabilised and complete closure was achieved.

At the end of surgery a long line was inserted into a central vein to allow for parenteral feeding later. The neonate remained intubated, was returned to the incubator and transferred back to the neonatal unit with positive pressure ventilation throughout. A morphine infusion was used to provide postoperative analgesia.

DISCUSSION POINTS

Gastroschisis develops as a result of occlusion of the omphalomesenteric artery during gestation. The consequence of this intrauterine vascular accident is an interruption in the abdominal musculature and subsequent herniation of intestinal contents.

- *Question 1:* *Given the pathogenesis of this defect, what are the likely associated anomalies?*

A major part of the anaesthetic care is directed towards measures to prevent hypothermia and continuing fluid resuscitation.

- *Question 2:* *How would you monitor the effectiveness of these manoeuvres?*

Exomphalos – although embryologically unrelated, and a more frequent anomaly – is managed surgically and anaesthetically in a similar manner to gastroschisis.

● **Question 3:** *What additional pre-operative investigation should be performed?*

Care was taken in the present case to place all monitoring equipment and intravenous lines in the upper half of the body.

● **Question 4:** *Why is this important?*

Respiratory and cardiac embarrassment were alluded to in the text.

● **Question 5:** *What other postoperative complications are highly likely?*

● **Question 6:** *When complete closure of the defect is not possible, what method is used to cover the defect?*

FURTHER READING

Gastroschisis. In: Stahling L, ed. Common problems in paediatric anaesthesia. St Louis. Mosby – Year Book, 1992; 19–25
Yaster M, Buck J R, Dudgeon D L et al. Haemodynamic effects of primary closure of omphalocoele/gastroschisis in human newborns. Anesthesiology 1988; 69: 84–88

Mollit D L, Ballantyne T V N, Grosfeld J L, Quin R P. A critical assessment of fluid requirements in gastroschisis. J Paed Surg 1978; 13: 217–219

De Vireos P A. The pathogenesis of gastroschisis and omphalocoele. J Paed Surg 1980; 15: 245–251

Roberts J D, Todores I D, Cote C J. Neonatal emergencies. In: Cote C J, Ryan J F, Todres I D, Goudsouzian N G, eds. A practice of anaesthesia for infants and children. 2nd ed. Philadelphia: WB Saunders, 1993: 240–242

James I G. Emergencies in paediatric anaesthesia. In: Sumner F, Hatch D J, eds. Textbook of paediatric anaesthetic practice. London: Balliere Tindall, 1989: 443–459

45 Cleft palate

A 9-month-old boy weighing 8.5 kg presented for repair of cleft palate. He was diagnosed as having Pierre Robin syndrome at birth. The plastic surgeon's normal practice was to operate on babies with cleft palate at 6 months. In this case, he allowed a little extra time for mandible growth, knowing that this condition is associated with difficulty in tracheal intubation.

The infant was born at 38 weeks by elective caesarean section for cephalopelvic disproportion. Because airway and feeding problems were anticipated, he was initially observed in the neonatal unit. Following an early apnoeic episode, the infant was nursed prone and the insertion of a nasopharyngeal airway was required to relieve the airway obstruction. Attempts at oral feeding resulted in further breathing difficulties, and a cyanotic episode and nasogastric feeding, was commenced. The oropharyngeal airway remained in situ for 3 weeks and nasogastric feeding continued for a further month. Despite the propensity for aspiration and chest infection, these complications were largely avoided, and the child continued to thrive.

On admission the boy was well with no evidence of infection. He appeared well-nourished and there were no abnormalities detected on examination of the cardiovascular or respiratory systems. The presence of micrognathia, an element of glossoptosis and a cleft palate were observed. The haemoglobin level was 12 g/dl and one unit of blood had been cross-matched.

Following oral premedication with atropine, anaesthesia was induced with oxygen, nitrous oxide and halothane. An indwelling venous cannula was inserted and an ECG and oxygen saturation monitor attached. A clear airway was maintained throughout, and it proved possible to ventilate the lungs manually using the face mask. Laryngoscopy was carried out under deep halothane anaesthesia and only the epiglottis could be seen. A size-two laryngeal mask airway (LMA) was inserted and a clear airway obtained. A gum elastic bougie was then passed through a hole in the rubber bung of the angle piece and gently placed through the LMA until it entered the trachea. A fibre-optic bronchoscope (external diameter 1.5 mm) was also passed to confirm the position of the bougie in the trachea. Anaesthesia was maintained throughout by spontaneous respiration of oxygen and halothane. The bronchoscope was withdrawn and then the LMA removed, taking care not to dislodge the bougie. A size 4.0 mm endotracheal tube was then rail-roaded over the bougie and the bougie removed. Following confirmation of the position of the tube by auscultation and end-tidal carbon dioxide measurement, atracurium was administered and mechanical ventilation of the lungs commenced with a mixture of 65% nitrous oxide and 0.5% isoflurane.

Surgery proceeded uneventfully, and a tongue stitch was placed prior to extubation. Isoflurane was discontinued and neuromuscular blockade was reversed. The infant was extubated when fully awake and, following a satisfactory period of observation in the recovery room, was transferred to the ward.

DISCUSSION POINTS

• *Question 1:* *What preparations would you make for the possibly difficult intubation of an infant?*

• *Question 2:* *The Pierre Robin syndrome occurs once in 50,000 births with an associated cleft palate in 50%. What other congenital abnormalities may be present, and how should they be screened for?*

• *Question 3:* *What are the long-term consequences of the upper airway obstruction which occurs in Pierre Robin syndrome?*

● **Question 4:** *The surgical site is generally infiltrated with local anaesthetic containing adrenaline. What are the recommended doses in an infant?*

● **Question 5:** *What problems might be encountered postoperatively, and what measures should be taken to avoid them?*

● **Question 6:** *What method of analgesia is most suitable for a child of this age having this type of surgery?*

FURTHER READING

Howardy-Hansem P, Berthelsen P. Fibreoptic bronchoscopic nasotracheal intubation of a neonate with Pierre Robin syndrome. Anaesthesia 1988; 43: 121–122

Lynch M, Underwood S. Pulmonary oedema following relief of upper airway obstruction in the Pierre Robin syndrome: a consequence of early palatal repair? Br J Anaes 1991; 66: 391–393

Allison A, McCrory J. Tracheal placement of a gum elastic bougie using the laryngeal mask airway. Anaesthesia 1990; 45: 419–420

Hollinger I. Pierre Robin syndrome. In: Stehling L, ed. Common problems in paediatric anaesthesia. St Louis: Mosby – Year Book, 1992, 63–68

Ward C T. Paediatric head and neck syndromes. In: Katz J, Steward D J, eds. Anaesthesia and uncommon paediatric diseases. 2nd edn. Philadelphia: WB Saunders, 1993: 319–363

Dykes E H, Raine P A M, Arthur D S, Drainer I K, Young D G. Pierre Robin syndrome and pulmonary hypertension. J Paed Surg 1985; 1: 49–52

Freeman M K, Manners J M. Cor pulmonale and the Pierre Robin anomaly. Anaesthesia 1980; 35: 282–286

46 Croup

A previously healthy 2-year-old girl was sent to hospital by her general practitioner with a diagnosis of croup. The medical senior house officer saw the child briefly in the Accident and Emergency Department and noted that her respiration was not unduly laboured with minimal stridor. Arrangements were made for her transfer to the medical ward for mist therapy and observation.

After several hours, the staff nurse caring for the child suspected that her breathing was deteriorating and attached a pulse oximeter which revealed an arterial oxygen saturation of 94% on air. The senior house officer was called, established venous access, and commenced intravenous rehydration and oxygen therapy. With oxygen, the child's arterial oxygen saturation increased to 97%. Paracetamol was prescribed for the child's pyrexia of 38.4°C.

Over the following 2 hours several episodes of desaturation occurred. The child's condition appeared to be deteriorating despite the mist therapy, oxygen and intravenous hydration, and nebulised adrenaline was administered. Racemic adrenaline was diluted and nebulised through a face-mask.

After an initial improvement in arterial oxygen saturation, the child's airway obstruction appeared to increase, with more marked indrawing. The arterial oxygen saturation continued to fall and the pulse rate slowed from 190/min to 75/min. Attempts to ventilate the child with a face mask were unsuccessful, and an emergency call was made for an anaesthetist.

Arriving on the ward three minutes later, the anaesthetist found a deeply cyanosed 2-year-old girl. The pulse oximeter displayed an arterial oxygen saturation of 52% and a pulse rate of 60/min. A face mask attached to a T-piece (Mapleson E circuit) was being held on her face, and she was making some inspiratory effort, but no air entry was evident. The anaesthetist lifted the mandible forcefully and opened the mouth of the child. Some movement of the T-piece bag was noted and the arterial oxygen saturation eventually started to rise. Not feeling very confident about managing this case single-handedly on the ward, the anaesthetist asked for senior assistance and transferred the child to the nearby operating theatre. Induction of anaesthesia was undertaken with halothane in oxygen and the arterial oxygen saturation had reached 90% on oxygen and 2% halothane when the consultant paediatric anaesthetist arrived in theatre. As the halothane concentration was gradually increased, the child's airway obstruction increased and the consultant decided to intubate the trachea.

Direct laryngoscopy was performed, and after copious secretions were removed by suction, the cause of the obstruction was visualised. A grossly swollen, bright red epiglottis was overlying the glottic aperture. A 4.5 mm nasotracheal tube was passed without difficulty and taped securely to the face. The signs of airway obstruction resolved immediately, although the respiratory rate remained rapid and the child was transferred to the intensive care unit.

DISCUSSION POINTS

Children with acute upper airway obstruction may exhibit an extremely rapid deterioration and the seriousness of their condition may not be fully appreciated. Whatever the cause of the obstruction, certain steps should be taken immediately.

- *Question 1: Can you describe a protocol for the management of these cases?*

- *Question 2: What features in the presenting history might have suggested that the diagnosis was not laryngotracheobronchitis?*

- *Question 3: The narrow diameter of paediatric endotracheal tubes renders them more liable to blockage with secretions etc. What steps would you take to avoid this?*

Other complications may develop despite relief of the obstruction. After intubation, frothy secretions were seen to issue from the endotracheal tube. These persisted despite repeated suction and the arterial oxygen saturation fell.

- *Question 4:* *What is the mechanism of the development of pulmonary oedema in this situation, and what treatment would you suggest?*

FURTHER READING

Mauro R D, Poole S R, Lockhart C H. Differentiation of epiglottitis from laryngotracheitis in the child with stridor. Am J Diseases of Childhood 1988; 142: 679–682

Blackstock D, Adderley R J, Steward D J. Epiglottitis in young children. Anesthesiology 1987; 67: 97–100

Molteni R A. Epiglottitis: incidence of extra-epiglottic infection. Report of 72 cases and review of the literature. Paediatrics 1976; 58: 526–531

Soliman M G, Richer P. Epiglottitis and pulmonary oedema in children. Can Anaesthetists Soc J 1978; 25: 270–275

47 Drowning

A 4-year-old boy was transferred to the Casualty Department approximately 30 minutes after an immersion injury in a neighbour's swimming pool. The history from his friend is that he slipped and fell into the shallow end of the pool. He was removed from the pool three to four minutes later by an adult with some training in basic life support who managed to clear the airway and ventilate the child by the mouth-to-mouth method. It was reported that at no time was the child without a pulse, although it had been slow and irregular when first felt. The ambulance team reported that the rescuer estimated that the child's first spontaneous gasp occurred within 'a couple of minutes' of initiating mouth-to-mouth ventilation.

On arrival, the child was drowsy and cried when stimulated. He felt cold, and peripheral perfusion was poor. There was no obvious evidence of bone fractures. Oxygen was administered by face-mask, ECG monitoring was established and his blood pressure was measured. Rectal temperature was recorded at 34.2°C. The electrocardiogram showed sinus tachycardia and his blood pressure was recorded as 70/40 mmHg.

Passive and external active rewarming measures were instituted. His wet clothing was completely removed and replaced with warm blankets. A warming mattress was placed around him on the trolley and intravenous dextrose – saline solution was administered through an infusion warmer. Arterial blood gas measurements are shown in Table 1. Blood was taken for serum electrolytes, glucose and blood cultures. A chest radiograph showed no abnormal pulmonary appearances.

Two hours later the boy was less drowsy and responded to questions. Rectal temperature had risen to 35.3°C and peripheral perfusion was improving. While a second arterial sample was being taken, the boy suddenly vomited a large volume of swallowed water. He was quickly turned onto his side and suction was used to clear his mouth. Despite the

Table 1 Blood results

	On admission: breathing air	2 hours later: breathing oxygen
pO$_2$ (kPa)	12.1	9.5
pCO$_2$ (kPa)	4.9	7.2
pH	7.26	7.30

rapid response, his respiratory pattern changed with obvious sub-costal indrawing and an increased respiratory rate. He was considerably less responsive, and it was feared that he may have aspirated some of the vomitus.

A second chest radiograph was ordered, and intravenous cefotaxime was administered. The chest radiograph showed no significant change compared with the previous film and no evidence of aspiration, however the arterial blood gas measurements showed a significant fall in pO_2 and a rise in pCO_2 (see Table 1). The child was transferred to the intensive care unit for further close observation and further management.

DISCUSSION POINTS

Immersion injuries are a leading cause of mortality in children. In the UK the annual incidence of immersion events has been reported as 1.5 per 100 000, with a mortality of 0.7 per 100 000, while in the USA drowning is the fourth leading cause of death for children under 19 years and the leading cause of death from injury for those under 5 years of age. In the UK 83% of these children were unsupervised at the precise time of the incident. The mortality from events in rivers, canals and private pools far exceeds that from events in public pools, probably due to different levels of supervision and ability to provide basic life support.

- *Question 1:* *What do the terms drowning and near-drowning convey?*

Rapid restoration of oxygenation and cerebral blood flow is obviously essential if there is a possibility of survival following an immersion event.

- *Question 2:* *Bearing in mind that victims may have swallowed significant volumes of water during an immersion and may have suffered other injuries, describe the early management of the patient with an immersion injury, both at the scene of injury and in the resuscitation room.*

● *Question 3: Was the management of this case optimal?*

● *Question 4: Which factors in the history are important in predicting outcome from an immersion event?*

There are dramatic case reports of survival after immersion events in icy water. These survivors have been in freezing water (< 5°C) with core temperatures of less than 28–30°C. Cold water drowning such as the one described above do not offer the protection occasionally seen with icy water, and hypothermia itself can produce multiple-system dysfunction. Restoration of normal temperature is important to optimise recovery.

● *Question 5: Why are children at high risk of hypothermia?*

● *Question 6: Discuss the options available for rewarming the hypothermic patient.*

FURTHER READING

Advanced paediatric life support: the practical approach. BMJ Publishing, 1993: 175–8

Kemp A M, et al. Outcome in children who nearly drown; a British Isles study. BMJ 1991; 302: 931–3

Fields A I. Near drowning in the pediatric population. Crit Care Clin 1992; 8: 113–129

Kemp A, Sibert J R. Drowning and near-drowning in the United Kingdom: lessons for prevention. BMJ 1992; 304: 1143–1146

Corneli H M. Accidental hypothermia. J Pediatrics 1992; 120: 617–679

Hastings R H, Marks J D. Airway management for trauma patients with potential cervical spine injuries. Anes Analg 1991; 73: 471–482

Index